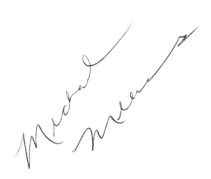

MW01251538

# ALSO BY MICHAEL MEIERS

*Was Jonestown a CIA Medical Experiment?*
*A review of the Evidence, 1989.*

# The Second HOLOCAUST

## How the AIDS Epidemic was Created in a CIA Black Operation

by
Michael Meiers

First published by Dog Ear Publishing
4010 W. 86th Street, Ste H
Indianapolis, IN 46268
www.dogearpublishing.net

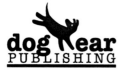

ISBN: 978-1-4575-2503-2

This book is printed on acid-free paper.

Printed in the United States of America

**"Those who do not remember the past are condemned to relive it."**

"...Maybe we should stop these 'niggers' and 'riff-raff' from terrorizing our neighborhoods, driving down property values, eating up our tax-payer's dollars on Welfare checks, spreading crime, drugs, and mayhem, corrupting our children... maybe send them all back to Africa or just get RID of them somehow, as Hitler rid Germany of the Jews and all other minorities."

"...Imagine that a military power, in pursuit of global conquest, could pinpoint genetic differences between the races and design chemical agents to ATTACK AND VIRTUALLY DESTROY ETHNIC OR RACIAL GROUPS!!!! Science fiction, you say? On the contrary, the creation of ETHNIC WEAPONS presents a terrifying present day threat."

Excerpts from Jim Jones's *People's Forum* published in San Francisco a few years before he fulfilled his own prophecy.

# DEDICATION

This book is dedicated to Congressman Leo Ryan's attorney and long time friend Joseph Holsinger without whose help and encouragement, the truth may never have been revealed. There were scores of others who helped me on my way, but it was Joe Holsinger who set me on the path. Back in 1980, in his Foster City, California living room, he helped lay the foundation for this and my previous book and assured me that I was not the only one who believed the CIA had killed a congressman. He accurately predicted that the pursuit would dominate my life, but I only wish that he had reminded me of the Chinese philosopher, Confucius, who wrote, " Before you embark on a journey of revenge, first dig two graves."

# CONTENTS

# THE PREFACE

*"The evil men do lives after them; the good is oft interred with their bones."*

—**William Shakespeare.**

I was the last person to speak with William Colby about his work, as the director of the Central Intelligence Agency, and he may have been killed for what he told me.

It was April 24th, 1996, and I had just sat through Mr. Colby's rather boring lecture at a local community college. I was standing in the corner at the reception that followed, waiting to ask him a few critical questions. The crowd had dwindled and the evening was drawing to a close, when he approached me. After exchanging a few pleasantries, I asked, "What difference did the Hughes-Ryan Amendment make in the operation of the Company?" Despite the late hour, Colby's eyes lit up and he became very animated. He was obviously excited to discuss what was at the heart of his tenure at the CIA. "Fundamental difference! Fundamental difference!", he exclaimed. "Why, I remember the first time I had to go into *that room* and tell Ryan what we were doing in Angola." Trying hard to maintain my composure, I asked, "Were we training mercenaries in the jungles of Guyana to fight in Angola?" Colby responded, "I can't say." Not satisfied, I asked, "Is it that you can't say because you don't know or is it that you can't say because you are not allowed to say?" Again he said, "I can't say." I pressed harder. "Did the agency resent Congressman Ryan for meddling in its affairs?" His only answer was, "I can't say."

Just then, we were interrupted by the event planner, who said, " Mr. Colby, it's time to go." Colby was driven to a motel near the Rochester International Airport where, the next morning, he boarded a flight to Washington, D.C. As for me, I drove home deep in thought. Colby couldn't have known who I was or the damage he had just done. Anyone else would consider our conversation to be innocent: anyone that is, but me. Eight years earlier, I had written a scholarly history entitled: *Was Jonestown a CIA Medical Experiment?* In it I documented the CIA's training of Brazilian mercenaries that were sent to fight in the CIA's war in Angola. They had been recruited by a promising young CIA operative operating in Belo Horizonte, Brazil in the early 1960's, named Jim Jones. The mercenaries were trained and equipped in a remote camp deep in the Guyana jungle that was later known as "The Jonestown Agricultural and Medical Project." As will be apparent later, it was eventually the site of CIA experiments in mind control and a field test in the communicable aspects of the AIDS virus, culminating in the largest "mass suicide" in history and the killing of Leo Ryan, the only US Congressman ever to be assassinated. When Colby told me that Ryan's first introduction into CIA black operations was Angola, I was ecstatic. For the first time, I understood that Ryan *knew* he was walking into a CIA project when he decided to investigate Jonestown, but he could not tell his aides, attorney, or anyone else who did not have the required security clearances. I had been studying the story from the bottom up and now the former director of the CIA was meeting me exactly in the middle from the top down. I was more convinced than ever that the CIA had killed Congressman Ryan.

The Hughes-Ryan Amendment of 1974 would have ultimately transferred oversight of the CIA from the president and the military to eight committees of Congress. Senator Harold Hughes and Representative Leo Ryan were reacting to President Nixon's use of the air force and navy in covert bombings of Cambodia and Laos during the Vietnam War. Presidents do not have the legal authority to conduct a war without Congress's approval. Furthermore, they questioned whether one man could grasp the enormity and complexity of the CIA's covert operations. There were accusations that the CIA were conducting operations without even informing the president. The first phase of the amendment's passage into law guaranteed Congressman Ryan unprecedented access to the nation's top secrets and he proceeded to badger the agency for information. The CIA **hated** Ryan. For thirty years they had operated with impunity and without accountability. Even their budget was a secret. Oversight by one of their own was bad enough, but they certainly were not going to tolerate oversight by an outsider; especially a loose cannon like Ryan. After his initial meetings with Colby, Ryan leaked a partial story of the CIA's involvement in Angola to newsman Daniel Schorr and the resulting expose' was a major embarrassment to the CIA for several months.

Ryan's murder in Guyana was first reported over a secret CIA frequency radioed from Jonestown. The CIA then phoned Ryan's attorney, Joe Holsinger, with the news. When Holsinger pressed the agent as to how he knew, he admitted, "We had an agent present."

I knew all this and volumes more when I first shook hands with William Colby and asked him that very loaded question about the Hughes-Ryan

Amendment. Our conversation was one of many such validating revelations that had occurred since the publication of my first book. Most disturbing was the reaffirmation that the medical hospital in Jonestown was studying the communicable aspects of the AIDS virus. Jonestown self-destructed one month before the first reported case of AIDS, and there is hard evidence to support that it was ground zero for the epidemic.

The timing for my first book was accidentally impeccable. Ten years after the fact, I was able to take advantage of all of the first hand accounts. They were surprisingly consistent in detail, but lacked the overview I provided by combining them into a comprehensive history. My research was old school; pre-Internet; one hard fought fact after another. The book is over 600 pages of names, dates, places, and photos that are accurate, but extremely tedious in detail and difficult to read. It was well received by a small group of scholars, historians, and those few individuals willing to pay the publisher's $175 cover price, but it was never intended for the general public. I did gain an international reputation as the curator of the finest library on the subject of Jonestown (outside of the CIA's). Whenever the *BBC, NBC,* or other media wanted to produce a feature story, they would contact me for background information. Occasionally, they borrowed books or documents that were out of print. Each used me for reference data, but their finished products always fell short of the truth. Typically, they agreed with me in private, but claimed they could not publish my findings out of concern for the feelings of the relatives of the dead. I think they were just afraid. Ultimately, the task of documenting the truth fell to me and I was looking forward to the challenge.

The next day at work, I could not get thoughts of the night before or a second book out of my mind. Traveling alone, Colby was making his way to his riverfront home in southern Maryland, where eventually he ended up. Colby loved this place. It was an old fisherman's crab shack when he bought it. He had put his heart and soul into renovating it into a modest but comfortable, retirement home for him and his wife. He arrived to an empty house, his wife was away visiting relatives. According to the accepted story, he left his half-eaten dinner on the table, walked down to the river in the dark, got into his canoe, paddled out into rough water, and drowned, but there were no witnesses. The next day, a neighbor called 911 after she found his canoe, but could not find him. A search crew of dozens, including several divers, did not discover his body until eight days later. The federal government was noticeably silent, relegating the investigation to the local authorities. The press immediately suspected foul play, if only because of his former position as director of the CIA and to some extent their suspicions were confirmed by the details. The coroner could not determine a definitive cause of death. They assumed drowning, but there was not enough water in his lungs to support that. Colby had a plaque build-up on some arteries, so they considered a heart attack or stroke, but they never checked for toxins that might have induced that, besides, too much time had passed to confirm either. In the end, they more or less threw up their hands in defeat and declared that it was an "accidental downing" based not on the body, but on the circumstances.

Why would Colby abandon his dinner to take a canoe trip in the dark in rough water? When they found the canoe, it was beached, upright, and full of sand— unlikely to have happened naturally, but understandable if someone did not want it to float away. Reportedly, it took the better part of an hour to scoop out the sand in order to tow the canoe away, but conveniently, there was already a tow line attached to the bow. After an exhausting week searching, the authorities retired Sunday afternoon, only to easily locate the body the following Monday morning. The body was found near the shoreline only 100 feet from the canoe in an area they had searched over and over again. It was just off the end of an isolated dirt road. It appeared as if Colby's body had been dumped there. His internal organs were too deteriorated for any objective autopsy, but his body was in as pristine a condition as a corpse could be. It showed absolutely no signs of being in the water for nine days. The only facts known with certainty are that Colby interrupted his dinner, disappeared, and was found dead in the water nine days later. Everything else was speculation. It is just as likely that Colby's dinner was interrupted by a knock at his door. He was abducted and murdered, the canoe was staged, and after sufficient time had passed to prevent the authorities from determining an accurate cause of death, the body was dumped back at the scene.

I was devastated when I heard the news. Colby should never have revealed even the subject matter of a top secret debriefing with Congressman Ryan. He should have turned on his heels and walked away when I asked about the Hughes-Ryan Amendment, but he was too polite, or my question was too intriguing, or maybe his guard was down when I said, "The Company," a phrase only insiders use to describe the CIA. Was he killed for a slip of the tongue to the wrong person? He was already in serious trouble with the agency for talking too much. In 1976, as the Guyana project was about to transition from a mercenary training camp to the Jonestown medical experiments, President Ford fired Colby from his top position at the CIA for "telling Congress too much about their clandestine operations." Given the timing and the characters involved, what President Ford was really saying was that Colby was telling Ryan too much about the Angola Project and Jonestown. Colby then used his retirement to write a book that prompted a lawsuit from the CIA, because he had disclosed even more classified information. Not wanting the publicity, they settled out of court and Colby paid a $10,000 fine. Since then, I am certain his activities, especially public appearances, like college lectures, were closely monitored.

William Colby was too much of a gentleman to live among wolves. He was honest, but talked too much. He was a security threat to the CIA in the past, the present, and they assumed that he would continue to be in the future. It was costing the agency more money to monitor his lectures than Colby was being paid for them. They had visions of chasing him from one community college to the next for years to come. My brief conversation with Colby was not important to anyone but me. To the CIA, it was just a straw, but it was the last straw. That night they decided he had to be eliminated, and even how.

The morning after the lecture, the event planner arrived at his college job to find a typed envelope on his desk. It was addressed to him and marked 'Personal and Confidential.' He later gave me a photocopy that reads:

"Dear Ray,

Thanks for the nice time at Finger Lakes.
I enjoyed it very much.
If you'd like to book a return engagement,
it'll have to wait awhile as I am planning an
underground (or is it underwater) assignment with
my old department. Anyway...they'll take care of me
I'm sure!
Cyanide...er sayanora?!
Your Friend,

Wm. Colby"

The note was signed, but the signature did not match the signature Colby had given the event planner, as a thank you note on a copy of the lecture announcement. It was obviously written by another hand.

Are we to believe that Colby was psychic, to predict his own death a few days later when he typed, 'or is it underwater'? and then there was the all too appropriate reference to "cyanide." Why would Colby risk telling an acquaintance that he was going "undercover" when, by doing so, it would be a breach of national security before his assignment even began? Why would a successful Washington lawyer, international consultant, author and lecturer, in good heath and spirits, need anyone to "take care" of him? In what context was that sentence written?

The purpose of the note was precisely its results. The event planner was convinced that Colby was in the CIA's good graces and was discouraged from contacting him during the next few critical days. After news reports of Colby's death, he was too frightened to speak out, though he did make one phone call to offer a copy of the note to help in the investigation. His call was never returned. They did not care about the note and, why should they, if they had written it.

William Colby's untimely death resurrected the fear, intrigue, and bizarre coincidences that had plagued my initial research. I continued studying and gathering data, but put this second book on hold for the next seventeen years while I tried to live a normal, quiet life. I knew that anyone who got too close to this story ended up with a bullet in the brain and I was closer than most, but I have reached that age when my days are growing short and looking back over my life, I have but one regret— not publishing this book earlier. In the words of Congressman Ryan on the eve of his trip to Guyana, "You have to put fear aside and do what you think is right."

As of today, over 35 million people have died from the AIDS epidemic and even more have been infected. I do not claim to have a cure, but what I do have is the cause and somewhere within that cause, there may be a cure.

This story has its roots in the early 1960s. Almost every major US city is ablaze. Race riots claimed hundreds of lives and inflicted millions of dollars in property damage. We know it now as the beginning of the Civil Rights Movement, but at the time, it had all the earmarks of the beginning of a Civil Race War. The CIA does not play catch up. They anticipate with 'what if' contingency plans. What if *this* happened, what would they do? What if *that* happened, what would they do? In this case; how could they control a rebellious black population? There were several possible solutions and one of them was pharmacutical.

# O N E

## OPERATION PAPERCLIP

*"Leaving Nazi scientists in Germany to be recruited by the Soviets would have presented a far greater threat to this country than any former Nazi affiliations they may have had or even any Nazi sympathies which they may still have."*

**—Bosquet Wev, Head of the U.S. Joint Intelligence Objectives Agency.**

Towards the end of World War II in Europe, US and British troops were advancing through Germany from the West, while our Soviet allies were advancing from the East. Tensions arose the moment the two invading forces met. The Soviets accused the US of stealing Hitler's gold. The US accused the Soviets of the same. Immediately our ally became our enemy. General George Patton attempted to get to the bottom of the problem, but was killed trying. It seems ludicrous now but, at the time, no one suspected that the Nazis had pirated away their own gold and had successfully pulled off a very simple 'divide and conquer' strategy that initiated the Cold War.

During World War II, the Soviets were our friends, so there was no need to gather intelligence on their activities. But after the war, we were blindsided by a new enemy that we knew nothing about. That intelligence void was filled when Reinhard Gehlen surrendered to US troops and offered his services. Gehlen was a master Nazi spy who controlled hundreds of deep cover operatives in the Soviet Union. He offered the US four steamer trunks full of sensitive, top secret Soviet documents and a network of spies and we could not refuse.

Previously, US intelligence gathering was the job of the Overseas Strategic Services. OSS agents were typically privileged academics who cabled their observations to the assistant librarian at Yale University. His expertise was indexing and he painstakingly referenced and cross referenced thousands of reports that were then available to the military, or the president, or anyone else with the proper clearances. The OSS was a gentlemen's club that believed that "Gentlemen do not read other gentlemen's mail," They were much too naive to survive in the brutal, post-war era. The OSS was disbanded. Some of its employees were folded in with the new Nazi intelligence network to consecrate an unholy marriage that we know today as the Central Intelligence Agency.

Following the US Army's march through Germany was a military group whose sole mission was to apprehend all Nazi doctors, researchers, and scientists and take them into custody to concentration camps called "dust bins," where they awaited their fate. Those with little to offer, were tried as war criminals. Those with more to offer, were pirated to the United States. The Nazi scientists had tried to position themselves to be captured by the Americans and not the Soviets. The Soviets were brutal. Their orders were, "Do not count miles, do not count time, count the number of Germans you have killed"- not just German soldiers, but any and all Germans were exterminated on the Soviet's march to Berlin. On the eve of their arrival in Berlin, 5,000 city residents committed suicide rather than face the Soviets. Nazi scientists had the freedom of mobility to move west, where they were more likely to be captured by the Americans. Their technology was far superior to our own and we were afraid that if we did not bring them into the US, the Soviets would use them and their knowledge against us.

In 1945, President Harry Truman authorized "Operation Paperclip" so named because US visas were paper clipped to the Nazi scientist's files. In the first few years after the war, over 1,600 Nazi scientists were brought to the US. A few of them became famous, even revered. There was no such thing as a US space program- what the US had was a German space program. Without the rocketry expertise of Germans like Wernher von Braun, we never would have been able to land on the moon. Unfortunately, other Nazi paperclip scientists continued their work in bacteriological and viral warfare and some of them worked together to forward their own secret agenda. Then there was one scientist doctor who was so notorious, so valuable, so wanted, that the US could not risk harboring him in the United States, so they helped him escape to a safe distance away in South America. His name was Josep Mengele.

Dr. Josep Mengele was the medical director of the Auschwitz Concentration Camp. As many as five trains arrived at Auschwitz every day and thousands upon thousands of "sub-humans" were ordered out of the cattle cars to form a single file line to pass by Mengele. With a riding crop in hand, Mengele motioned each either to the right or to the left, to their immediate death in the gas chambers or a slow death slaving in the I.G. Farben factories. Sending thousands of innocent people to their deaths was not an easy task.

Medical directors at other concentration camps had to drink heavily just to live with the guilt, but not Mengele. Steely-eyed and sober, Mengele ordered the murder of hundreds of thousands of people, earning him the nickname, "The Angel of Death."

Mengele was obsessed with twins, both for experimentation and to unlock their secret in order to double the Aryan repopulation of the world, but his foremost expertise was in Tay-Sachs—"The Jewish Disease." His research had begun at the Third Reich Institute for Heredity, Biology and Racial Purity at the University of Frankfort where he was radicalized, joined the SS, and received his commission at Auschwitz. Tay-Sachs is a fatal autosomal recessive genetic disorder that effects only Jews of Eastern European descent. It is caused by a genetic defect in one gene that is inherited from both parents. Deterioration of mental and physical abilities first appear at six months of age and results in death before age four. Scientists believe that Tay-Sachs originated sometime in early history during what they call a 'population bottleneck'; a clinical description of inbreeding. There is no cure, but Mengele was not looking for a cure, he was looking to understand the cause, in order to replicate it as an ethnic weapon to be used against all Jews. There is a similar autosomal recessive genetic disorder called Sickle Cell Anemia that affects only people of African or Southern Mediterranean descent. By the early 1970s, the finest Sickle Cell Anemia clinic in the United States was run by upwards of seventy nurses who worked for Jim Jones.

With the Soviet Army quickly advancing from the west, Mengele abandoned his post at Auschwitz, packed up all of his blood samples, and traveled east to Gross Rosen, the site of Nazi biological weapons research. He collected the results of their experiments and continued onto the next laboratory. Mengele was on a mission to preserve all Nazi knowledge of biological and viral weaponry. Eventually, he met up with the Americans who first let him go. Mengele was so arrogant that he expected to continue his work in Europe, but that was obviously not possible. Recognizing the value of his information, the Americans brought him into Operation Paperclip and assured his passage, not to the US, but to South America.

Mengele was first harbored in Argentina, then Paraguay, and finally Brazil. He had established a pharmaceutical company that produced drugs, but only those used in his continued research. He moved from place to place, always just a step ahead of his Israeli pursuers who were trying to bring Mengele to justice for his crimes against Jews in Auschwitz. One time they were so close that Mengele had to flee his hotel room at 2 a.m., still wearing his pajamas. He was the most wanted man in the world and he was running out of options. His family back in Germany was very wealthy. Before the war, the Mengele's factory had manufactured farm equipment, but the largest share of their wealth came after the war when they made wheelbarrows that were used universally throughout Europe to clean up the bombed out rubble. By the early 1960s, Mengele's family had disowned him, and without their financial support, he was totally reliant on his CIA handlers, whose job was to extract all of his knowledge. Mengele had managed to stay alive by spoon-feeding them one insignificant fact after another, but the time had come for the CIA to demand everything. Jim Jones was a promising young operative working undercover nearby, who had an extraordinary ability to manipulate people, so they set up a meeting between Jones and Mengele. They hoped it would result in Mengele finally telling everything he knew, but what they might not have realized was that they were creating a monster that would eventually kill over 100 million people.

In addition to Gehlen's spies and the Paperclip scientists, there was one other Nazi element in the United States. Just like the Nazis had planted spies in the Soviet Union prior to the war, they had done the same here in the United States. One of these deep cover agents was Lisa Philip who had managed to marry the director of the US Army's Chemical and Biological Warfare Division. Once a week, for two years, Jim Jones spent almost an entire day at her home. Her daughter was one of Jim Jones's top aides, who supposedly defected from the Peoples Temple to convince Congressman Ryan to investigate Jonestown, while her son was the only person ever convicted for plotting to kill him.

Today, very little remains of the massive complex of the Auschwitz Concentration Camp. One gas chamber and one crematorium were preserved for posterity. There are a few remaining buildings and overgrown railroad tracks, but what stands out is the cast iron sign over the main gate, coined by the Nazi's Minister of Economics, Dr. Hyalmar Schacht, that reads, **"Work Shall Set You Free"**. The one doctor in Jonestown was Larry Schacht. When you enter the headquarters of the Central Intelligence Agency, you are greeted by a sign, carved in the marble wall that reads, **And Ye Shall Know The Truth and The Truth Shall Set You Free"**. Nothing about this story will set you free.

# T W O

## DEEP COVER

*"I.G. Farben was Hitler and Hitler was I.G. Farben"*

**—US Senator Homer Bone,**
**Senate Committee on Military Affairs.**

I.G. Farben was a huge German chemical trust and the engine that powered the Nazi's war machine. They provided the synthetic rubber, aviation fuel, explosives, and just about everything else the Nazi military needed. They helped to develop the vast network of concentration camps that provided free slave labor to produce the basic elements of their war machine. They even manufactured the Zyklon B gas to kill those who could not work. They made a fortune and entrusted that fortune to a Hamburg banker and stock broker named Hugo Philip.

While most Germans suffered under the financial burden of severely imposed World War I reparations, the Philips family fortunes increased exponentially. Hugo commissioned a renowned architectural firm to design and build his ultra-modern home that rivaled the finest in Germany. Hugo was a patron of the arts who amassed a huge collection of extremely valuable paintings. He had three passions: art, music, and mountain climbing. He was said to be the most accomplished amateur musician in Hamburg. Every Christmas and Easter, he would host lavish parties and entertain his guests playing his priceless violin, crafted by a student of Stradivarius; and his Steinway grand piano. Whether in peace or in war, every year of his life, Hugo traveled to Austria to climb the Alps. It was his sanctuary and later the sanctuary for vast fortunes that he had buried there. When his daughters Lisa and Eva were not in private schools, they were touring health spas in southern Germany, escorted by their mother Anita. The Philip family was truly the elite of Nazi Germany, but they had a secret avocation. They placed Nazi spies in the United States prior to the war and Nazi criminals after the war.

The first to go was Hugo's cousin, the eminent nuclear physicist Dr. James Franck. Dr. Franck had won the Nobel Prize in Physics in 1925 and by the late 1930s was of tremendous value to the Nazis, who were trying desperately to develop the atomic bomb. On the surface, it would seem ludicrous that Hitler would let him go, but he did. Dr. Franck immigrated to the United States and ultimately joined the Manhattan Project to help build the first atomic bomb. In retrospect, it was a smart move for the Nazis. German research had reached a standstill. With Dr. Franck embedded in the Manhattan Project, the Germans were able to piggyback on US research to speed up their own, but this meant only one thing— Dr. Franck was a Nazi spy.

Hugo's wife, Anita, volunteered with an organization whose stated purpose was to place German girls in positions of power throughout the world. In other words, she was placing Nazi spies under deep cover. Her daughter Lisa was one such subject.

In 1938, on the eve of World War II, Anita arranged for Lisa to immigrate to the US. They needed to provide immigration with a logical reason, so they claimed she was Jewish, but because there was no evidence to that effect, it did not work and she was denied. Hugo then joined a Jewish social club but never attended meetings, and let his membership expire as soon as Lisa was granted her immigration papers. Lisa left Germany with a passport stamped "Judah" and sailed to America, were she went to work at the Kingsington Settlement House in Philadelphia, an underground end-of-the-line safe house to help German Nazis acclimate to their new lives in America.

The target of Lisa and her uncle's mission was a brilliant, very promising young American scientist named Dr. Lawrence Layton. Dr. Layton's father had invented the electric circuit breaker that over 100 years later is still the industry standard. He then passed his intelligence and innovative thinking on to his son. Lawrence was so brilliant that he successfully completed a one year course in differential calculus in just two weeks. He was one of only three in his class of forty to earn his masters degree from West Virginia University, where he invented a molecular still that gained him international acclaim.

Dr. Layton continued his education at the main campus of Penn State University, because it had a reputation for excellence in chemistry and physics. Whether by chance or design, his professor was Dr. James Franck who not only required Layton to be proficient in German, but recommended his niece Lisa as his best tutor. Learning German is not easy, so Lawrence and Lisa needed to spend a lot of time together. Lisa was absolutely gorgeous, with a sultry beauty that rivaled the Austrian movie star Hedy Lamarr. She could have dated any man on campus, but she selected Lawrence, who was an unattractive introvert more concerned with his science than with people.

Lawrence wanted nothing to do with Lisa's advances. He just did not like her, but she had a mission and failure was not an option. Lisa had the quintessential personality of a Nazi. She was sanctimonious, self-righteous, domineering, and arrogant. As they walked about the campus of Penn State, she would deliberately alter her step to crush ants on the sidewalk. Lawrence asked why she did this and she replied, "I learned to hate weak things in Germany."

Lisa's pursuit of Lawrence was relentless, but Lawrence was not interested until Lisa struck a nerve. Lawrence had only one girlfriend in his life, Constance Jefferies, who he met early on at New River State College. They dated, but eventually grew apart. When the newspaper articles appeared about the brilliant young scientist who had invented a molecular still, Constance Jefferies reportedly committed suicide. Lawrence always felt responsible, even guilty for her death, and Lisa knew it when she threatened to commit suicide if Lawrence didn't marry her. Not wanting another death on his conscience, Layton reluctantly agreed and they were married on October 18, 1941. They had known each other for only six months. Three weeks later, the Japanese attacked Pearl Harbor and we entered World War II.

As soon as the Laytons were married, Dr. Franck went to work at the University of Chicago on the Manhattan Project to develop the atomic bomb. He arranged for Dr. Layton to receive a military deferment, with an appointment to the project that would use his molecular still to purify uranium isotopes for the first atomic bomb.

Dr. Layton was appointed to a position at Eastman Kodak Company in Rochester, New York, were he continued to perfect his invention. On December, 2, 1942, the nuclear age was born when Dr. Franck, using Dr. Layton's purified uranium, set off the first self-sustaining nuclear reaction in a makeshift laboratory under the grandstands of the University of Chicago's football field.

World War II was well under way and back in Germany, Hugo and Anita Philip were unexplainably allowed to sell their house and move all their priceless possessions to just over the Austrian border to Northern Italy, where they purchased a boarding house. According to the family's published cover story, Hugo and Anita were then arrested for being Jewish and put on a train bound for a concentration camp. This brings to mind a picture of cattle cars stuffed with hundreds of people, but Hugo and Anita had a suite next to the club car. Supposedly, they took poison that only made them sick so the engineer stopped the train to let them out to receive medical treatment at the Catholic hospital in Lienz, Austria. They stayed for a few days to "recuperate," but the Nazis never returned for them so they proceeded over the Brenner Pass to their new home in Italy. Continuing in the family business, the Philip home would be a safe house on what was called the "Rat Run," the exodus of Nazi criminals from Germany to the Americas. Fugitive Nazis made their way to that same Catholic hospital in Lienz, Austria where they were met by Hugo, who guided them on foot over the Brenner Pass to his boarding house in Italy. They were given food, shelter, new clothes, forged documents, and instructions on how to proceed to the Americas.

Meanwhile, back in the US, Dr. Franck and his German colleagues succeeded in perfecting the atomic bomb, but waited to make their announcement until two weeks after Germany had surrendered. Dr. Franck's contribution to Germany may not have been stealing the secrets of the bomb, but in preventing it from being used against his Fatherland.

In 1946, Dr. Layton accepted a position at Johns Hopkins University as a professor and researcher in biochemistry. He was hired by Reginald Archibald of the Rockefeller Institute of Medical Research to develop a procedure for diagnosing cartilaginous cancer. Today, research into cartilaginous cancer is synonymous with research into the HIV/ AIDS virus. This may be the first insight into the AIDS pandemic that would follow. Dr. Layton's findings were a major medical breakthrough and his subsequent report, published in medical journals in 1951, gained him a professional prestige he had not known since his invention of the molecular still. He was invited to lecture at universities in England, Switzerland, and Germany. While in Germany, he received a letter from the US Army, offering him twice his salary as the director of their Chemical and Biological Warfare Division which he accepted. The offer came out of the blue. It was very strange that they sent it to him, while he was on tour in Germany and not to his home in the US; it was almost as if his job interview was conducted in Germany.

In his new position, Dr. Layton oversaw the most advanced chemical, biological, and viral warfare laboratory in the world, at Fort Detrick, Maryland as well as the Plum Island Animal Disease Research Center and the Dugway Proving Grounds in Utah. Even today, the Russians claim that the HIV virus was created in his Fort Detrick lab, because, in addition to their work developing viral weapons, the facility is the foremost research center for AIDS. The Dugway Proving Grounds is one of the most desolate places on earth, with countless miles of hard packed sand and salt. Dr. Layton spent much of his time there trying desperately to deploy the Army's arsenal of chemical and biological weapons, but without much success. Farm animals were tethered in concentric circles and the pathogens were dropped from a tower or an airplane. The animals, some dead, some still alive, were then recovered and dissected to record the effect of the toxins. Dead was not good enough for Layton- he developed a test to determine just *how* dead an animal was. In his time with the Army, Layton invented only ten new toxins, but over one hundred new ways to deploy them. This ten to one ratio is important to explain Layton's contribution. He and his colleagues at Dugway joked that they were not germ warfare scientists, but meteorologists, because no matter how lethal the pathogen was, the wind just blew it away.

Layton's conclusion at Dugway was that germ warfare was good, but aerial deployment was bad, so he began researching other means to spread his poisons. Some of his new delivery systems were ingenious. A canister filled with a deadly agent was packed into a suitcase outfitted with an external atomizer. The plan was for an unwitting participant to carry the suitcase through an airport terminal and infect all the passengers and airline personnel, who would then board planes to their various destinations, where they would transmit the disease to the locals. It was about this time that Layton started experimenting on people. First there were the soldier volunteers at the Army's Edgewood Chemical and Biological Arsenal near Fort Detrick. Soldiers were promised weekends home with their families and other privileges in exchange for their participation as guinea pigs in Layton's experiments. Then Dr. Layton got very brazen and exploded germ warfare bombs in the subways of New York City and on the streets of San Francisco and several small communities in Florida. His scientists would track the results of the experiments by gleaning reports of deaths and illness from hospitals, doctors and clinics, but these attempts failed. The reporting was too piecemeal. There were just too many places a person could go for medical treatment, and some victims that fell ill did not seek any help. Layton repeated some experiments in Winnipeg, Canada, where socialized medicine provided one stop shopping for his results.

Back in Europe, all the "Nazi rats" had run the "Rat Run" and Hugo and Anita Philip's work was finished, freeing them to leave. They arrived in the US in the spring of 1952 and no explanation has ever been given for why they split up on the docks. Hugo reportedly went to Boston, while Anita ended up on the streets of Manhattan- literally. She fell from the window of a skyscraper above. Her death was ruled a suicide because someone had left a note behind that read:

"My friends , know that I, free and proper, am a good American. But I was a gossip and was entangled in a network of intrigue. I no longer have the strength to free myself from it. Forget me not my beloved children and family. And you, Hugo, forgive me. Live well. All of you loved mankind so well."

It is possible that Anita's death was a suicide, but that does not explain the "intrigue" that she was "entangled" in, nor does it explain how she could claim to be a "good American" when she had been in this country for only a few days. Hugo almost immediately returned to Germany; the spouse is always the prime suspect in a murder. More than likely, Anita was killed by her own people. She had outlived her usefulness and her transparent history was a threat to her daughter's deep cover and the primary mission that awaited her. As an ultimate irony, Anita had written her suicide note claiming to be a "good American," in German.

After two very productive years with the army, it was the navy's turn to utilize Layton's genius. A "friend" from Washington arranged for him to be appointed associate director of Research and Development at the Naval Powder Facility at Indian Head, Maryland. Supposedly, his work centered on arming the navy's intercontinental missiles and Vanguard satellites, but it was classified top secret, so it could have been anything. Layton spent four years with the navy and then moved to Berkeley, California where he accepted a position as research scientist with the US Department of Agriculture's Western Regional Research Laboratory. Even at the Department of Agriculture, his work was war related. He studied whether farm animals could be safely eaten after being exposed to nuclear radiation. According to an article in the **New York Times**, in 1961, "He (Dr. Layton) published a paper that outlined, for the first time, an effective way to use laboratory monkeys to test human food allergies; previously such research could only be done on humans." This would be Layton's last published contribution to science and rather ironic considering that his next project was a top secret, unpublished experiment using human subjects instead of lab monkeys in an experiment known as Jonestown.

Dr. Layton lived in the Berkeley Hills in what his family called "the mansion" and, yes, by now there was a family. Lawrence and Lisa had four children— the two eldest, Thomas and Annalisa, had little to do with this story, but the two youngest, Deborah and Larry, had everything to do with Jonestown.

Larry was like his father— quiet, reserved, not very social, and according to reports, ignored as an unwanted child. Deborah, on the other hand, was like her mother; a spitfire. Her later, more affluent upbringing bred a spoiled brat with a holier than thou attitude. She has been described in print as "spiteful, arrogant, devious, sharp-tongued, pissy and bitchy." She was the family's problem child. She was expelled from high school in her freshman year. The family moved her into her older sister's school district, where once again, she was expelled. They then moved her into her older brother's school district and again, she was expelled; though the school agreed to take her back if she underwent psychological counseling. With few options left, the Laytons sent Deborah to a military school in England, run by Quakers. She finished high school and returned with George 'Phil' Blakey, a young Englishman she had met there, but the arrangement seems to have been predetermined. Blakey came from a wealthy English family with substantial stock holdings in a subsidiary of I.G. Farben, but the real connection was that Blakey was an MI6 intelligence agent (the British equivalent to the CIA).

According to the family, the Laytons were first introduced to Jim Jones through Larry's wife Caroline Moore, whose father was the Methodist minister on the U. C. Davis campus, where Larry and Caroline lived; but this just does not make sense. Why would a minister recommend that his daughter and son-in-law join another church? It is likely that Dr. Layton or Lisa initiated the contact, but in any event, Larry and Carolyn joined Jones's Peoples Temple, pledged 25% of their income, and were quickly divorced. Some reports claim that Jones had sex with one or both of them. It was the era of the Vietnam War and the military draft was after Larry who had been denied several appeals for a conscientious objector status. His moral objections to war and killing were not sufficient grounds to exclude him from mandatory military service. Jim Jones offered to write a letter to the draft board, "guaranteed to result in C.O. status". Jones's letter succeeded in getting Larry a deferment. In all probability, he told them he was homosexual. Larry was required to do community service at the Mendocino State Hospital, where other Peoples Temple aides worked.

When Deborah Layton and Phil Blakey returned from England, they immediately joined Larry and the Peoples Temple. Lisa soon followed. Dr. Layton never got involved because Jones came to him every weekend, where they met in private in his Berkeley Hills home. Blakey's visa was running out, so Jones arranged for him to marry Deborah and stay in the US to complete his training. Deborah and Phil never lived together. Their marriage was a sham.

As described later, Jones played a large part in the transition of British Guiana into an independent Guyana. For financial reasons, the Brits were willing to give up their colony, but like the US, did not want it to fall into the hands of the communists who were positioned to take control. Everything after that was a joint operation between the CIA and MI6, so it was inevitable that MI6 agent George 'Phil' Blakey and Jim Jones join forces. Blakey was a sea captain, so Jones purchased an ocean going ship for him to transport his recruits. In 1973, Jones sent Blakey to Guyana with an advance team of nine or ten administers and two hundred former Green Beret Special Forces troops to carve a settlement out of the jungle and run the Shalom Project that would later be renamed, "The Jonestown Agricultural and Medical Project," or simply "Jonestown."

Dr. Layton had "tickets," which is insiders slang for security clearances. He needed them for his work. Lisa, on the other hand, was just a housewife, but she had managed to pass several security checks, while the federal government was checking into her husband, so she decided to put her few "tickets" to use. She went to work at U.C. Berkeley's library, where she was in charge of radical left-wing publications. She was a CIA reader, who read everything that passed over her desk and forwarded anything of interest onto the CIA. She also provided the agency with the names of every library card holder who requested this information. When she started in the late 1960s, Berkeley was a hot bed of political unrest and the CIA needed to monitor it, if not act on it.

Lisa followed her children into the Peoples Temple and started giving Jones large amounts of money. She gave him $250,000 in 1970s from the Layton family estate and more, after her divorce from Lawrence, and even more from her father's stash in the Austrian Alps. All this money needed to be accounted for, so her daughter, Deborah was put in charge of Jones's finances. Deborah managed the day to day accounting as well as researching international banking laws and traveling overseas to establish numbered accounts in dozens of countries where the money could be hidden.

It was the later half of 1978, the November deadline was quickly approaching, and it was time for the Layton family members to get into their respective positions. Dr. Lawrence Layton remained in his mansion never leaving to visit his family in Redwood Valley, San Francisco, or Guyana. The family reported that he stayed in communication with his wife and children by monitoring the short wave radio conversations from Jonestown through an old friend from his days with the army. The family named him Joe Ajax and said he relayed messages to Lawrence. Joe Ajax was a fictitious name to accompany a fictitious story. Jonestown radio communications were in code with predetermined frequency changes. If there was a Joe Ajax he had to know the CIA code. In all probability, it was Lawrence listening to his own radio in his mansion.

Lisa was living in Jonestown and, as the matriarch of the project, was treated like the queen. While the other residences were crowded 15 to 20 people per cabin, Lisa had a cabin all to herself. Unlike everyone else, she had no responsibilities, no job to do, except one— plan a graceful escape before November.

After a brief trip back to the US, Larry Layton returned to Jonestown with the community's new X-ray machine. Jones had sent Larry to Santa Rosa College to learn to be an X-Ray technician and now he had his own personal machine. It was used only twice; once to X-ray his mother Lisa's chest and once to X-Ray an elderly black women who was dying from pneumocystis carinrii pneumonia. Jones switched the names on the reports and rather than give them to his own Dr. Schacht or a hospital in Guyana, he sent them back to San Francisco so a US doctor would confirm that "Lisa Layton" was dying.

Deborah Layton returned to the US from Jonestown to write the "Affidavit of Deborah Layton Blakey Re: The Threat and Possibility of Mass Suicide by Members of The Peoples Temple." It was an eleven page, thirty-seven point outline that she sent to Secretary of State Cyrus Vance and Congressman Leo Ryan. It hit Ryan squarely between the eyes. Over a thousand of his constituents were in Guyana, in what William Colby had told him was a CIA operation, and now they were planning to kill themselves? Between the CIA and Deborah Layton, Ryan was confused, but completely intrigued, he had no choice, but to go see for himself.

About two weeks before the massacre, two things happened on the same day. Phil Blakey sailed out of the story and Lisa Layton disappeared. Blakey boarded the Albatross at Port Kaituma with a crew and passengers, who then made their way down the river, out into the open ocean, and onto stops in Port of Prince, Haiti, and Port of Spain, Trinidad. In the aftermath, only Blakey was reported to be on board, but certainly he would have needed a crew to get there. Who were these crew members or passengers? They have never been identified and for good reason. Some were homosexual followers of Jones who carried the AIDS virus to the gay houses of prostitution in Haiti. Another passenger was Lisa Layton. Lisa escaped just two weeks before the mass suicide that culminated the experiments she had helped to finance. News of her so-called "death" did not leave Jonestown. Jones only told his followers that Lisa had died. There was no funeral, burial, or gravesite. Her body has never been recovered. Everyone just took Jones's word for it. Larry was reportedly so despondent at the news of his mother's "death", that Jones increased his dosage of anti-psychotic drugs. Her family back in the states did not learn of Lisa's "passing" until after the massacre.

As Congressman Ryan prepared to leave Jonestown with his contingent of reporters and defectors, Larry left a huddle with Jones and announced that he, too, wanted to defect. The others objected, but Ryan accepted him into the group. At the airstrip, Larry immediately boarded one of the two planes to plant a gun. As the group assembled around the planes, CIA operative Dick Dwyer required all the passengers to be patted down for weapons. When Dwyer was convinced that they had no defense, the assault team at the end of the runway started shooting. Larry went back into the plane to retrieve his hand gun. He shot and wounded Jonestown defectors Monica Bagby and Vernon Gosney. He tried to shoot the pilot and defector Dale Parks, but his gun misfired and Parks was able to wrestle it from Larry's hand. Meanwhile, the assassin at the end of the runway approached and shot Congressman Ryan and several others. Larry was immediately arrested, but the man who murdered Ryan was allowed to leave.

You cannot kill a United States congressman without someone taking the fall for it, and Larry Layton was dubbed the scapegoat from the beginning. Larry was immediately arrested by Dwyer's bodyguards and charged with attempted murder for shooting Bagby and Gosney.

"I, Larry Layton, take full responsibility for all the deaths and injuries that took place at the Port Kaituma airstrip. I felt that these people were working in conjunction with the CIA to smear the Peoples Temple."

This was Larry's confession to the Guyanese authorities that would seem to be an open and shut case for immediate prosecution, but that did not suit the CIA, that wanted the story to be "old news" before it went to trial. Larry languished in a Guyana prison for seventeen months before being brought to justice. He was not tried for Ryan's death. That was under US jurisdiction. He was only tried for the attempted murder of Bagby and Gosney. The defense did not present any evidence or witnesses. Larry took the stand, but broke down in tears and said nothing. Despite ballistic evidence that proved the bullet in Vern Gosney came from Layton's gun, despite Gosney's testimony, despite a signed confession, Larry Layton was found **innocent**, but unexplainably sent back to prison for another six months. The CIA was stalling until Jonestown was "old news,"

Finally, Larry was extradited to the US, where in August of 1981, he appeared in the US District Court in San Francisco, charged with "conspiracy to assassinate Congressman Ryan." By now, nearly three years had passed and the whole episode was just a bad memory. The prosecutor was US attorney William Hunter, who we will see later worked with Jones's attorney, Tim Stoen, to cover up the election fraud perpetrated by Jones in the 1975 San Francisco elections. When this scandalous conflict of interest was disclosed, Hunter stepped down and appointed his assistant Robert Dordero as prosecutor.

Prosecuting attorney Robert Dordero called twenty-one witnesses, all of whom testified that Larry was a member of the assassination team. An FBI ballistics expert confirmed that the bullets removed from Bagby and Gosney came from Larry's gun. Defense attorney Tony Tamburello countered that his client probably did attempt to kill Bagby and Gosney, but had nothing to do with killing Ryan. It was a safe admission because Larry had already been acquitted of attempted murder in Guyana and double jeopardy prevented a retrial. Larry was only on trial for "conspiracy" to assassinate Ryan.

According to the local media reports, The defense claimed Larry was a "government scapegoat. "The State Department is responsible for a monumental tragedy, and what they were trying to do now was blame one individual and divert attention from their own responsibility." They claimed that Larry was drugged into participating and that he looked "spaced out and was mumbling of a CIA conspiracy" during the attack.

Dick Dwyer, Deputy Chief of Mission at the US Embassy in Guyana and veteran CIA operative, testified for the prosecution. He had witnessed the assault from only a few feet away. Defense attorney Tony Tamburello told Judge Peckham that he questioned Dwyer's motives and wanted to know if, in fact, Dwyer worked for the CIA. He said Dwyer's testimony was "tainted by bias." He wants Larry Layton convicted to take responsibility of Jonestown off the State Department and the CIA." Judge Peckham disallowed that line of questioning, but when asked of his CIA involvement outside the courtroom, Dwyer gave the standard Company response, " I can neither confirm nor deny the allegation." In a prepared statement to the press, Tamburello said, " We believe Mr. Dwyer is biased and has a motive for saying what he is saying because it takes the heat away from the State Department; and particularly the CIA."

Even prosecution witnesses alluded to a CIA conspiracy. Dale Parks, who had wrestled the gun from Larry at the airstrip, testified that Larry had told Dale's father that Dale was part of a CIA conspiracy to destroy Jim Jones. The irony is, while Larry's trial progressed with CIA this and CIA that, on the other side of the story, Congressman Ryan's daughter was suing the CIA for $63 million dollars for what she claimed was the agency's responsibility for her father's murder. Murderer or victim, prosecution or defense, everyone was claiming CIA involvement.

The defense rested without calling a single witness, just vague references to the CIA. Unbelievable as it is, the jury returned deadlocked; 11 to 1 **in favor of acquittal.** The judge declared a mistrial and "released Larry on a personal recognizance bond signed by the defendant's father; who court records say was a "a retired germ warfare scientist who lives in the East Bay."

Under pressure to resolve the assassination, the prosecution was forced to retry their scapegoat, but they allowed him to live free until February, 1982, however the proceedings were further postponed until September of 1984, while the Court of Appeals considered a request to admit further evidence of CIA involvement. Just prior to the scheduled court date, Larry elected to have polyps removed from his throat. The defense argued that their client could not testify, so again the trial date was postponed. Finally in March of 1987, over eight years after the fact, Larry was tried, convicted. and sentenced to life in prison. Judge Peckham did add a footnote that Larry would be eligible for parole in only five years because he was not "primarily responsible" for the killings.

Larry's defense aside, the Layton family as a whole needed an alibi for their actions so a public relations campaign was contrived to paint them as innocent victims, even though they had as much to do with the Jonestown experiment as did Jim Jones. First there were well placed newspaper articles on both the east and west coasts. The **New York Times** carried an in-depth, front page article entitled, "The Layton Family Tragedy: From Hitler's Germany to Jim Jones' Commune." It was intended to play well with the New York City Jewish population. It described the family as having "a proud family tradition of Quaker nonviolence, a far cry from the reality that Dr. Layton's work was to create new ways to kill vast numbers of people, but such was the family's desperate attempts to distance themselves from the carnage they had created. They took a slightly different approach on the west coast with an article that appeared in the **San Francisco Chronicle**: "How the Temple Shattered a Family", in which they described a broken man, bewildered by what had befallen his family. He was described as a "molecular biologist and chemist" with a pacifist Quaker upbringing. The article never mentioned that he worked to create biological weapons of mass death, only that he "cried easily."

A very strange book came next. The Layton's eldest child, Thomas, was not involved in the Peoples Temple. He was studying at U.C. Davis earning his degree, then onto Harvard for his post-graduate work in anthropology. Thomas published a book entitled, *In My Father's House: The Story of the Layton Family and the Reverend Jim Jones,* that he co-authored with Min Yee, a professional writer. The book is worth reading for the history of the family, but it is peppered with Thomas's very strange observations. He admits that the CIA was a common topic of conversation in the Layton household, but fails to tell whether those conversations were pro or con. He implies that his entire family was homosexual. He wrote that his father was raised as a girl, in dresses and bobbed hair, who matured with no interest in women. Of his mother, he wrote that she had learned that everyone was homosexual and that she had probably been homosexual all her life. He said that she asked her daughter if Tom was as well, adding that some of her best friends were gay. Thomas even published a letter Deborah had allegedly written to Phil Blakey, but never mailed, in which she asked Blakey if homosexuality made him feel incapable? Thomas claimed that Jim Jones broke up Larry's first marriage to Carolyn Moore, when Jones had sex with Larry.

Though the concept of an entire family of homosexuals is contrary to the accepted science that sexual preference is not a matter of heredity, the real question is not whether the Laytons were a family of homosexuals, but why Thomas would go out of his way to imply that they were? Considering that they were working to create a plague to destroy all homosexuals, implying that they were homosexual was a defense. It was not a good defense or grounded in any fact, but it was their only defense.

Ultimately, Dr. Layton died in his Berkeley Hills mansion. Lisa was God only knows where; perhaps back with her father in Germany. Phil Blakey returned to his work in Angola, Africa. Deborah took a job as a money manager in the financial district in San Francisco. Thomas was a professor of anthropology at San Jose State University and the unwanted child, Larry, was in prison.

# T H R E E

## IN THE BEGINNING...

*"Stay calm. Do not let emotions, like anger, cloud your judgment. Approach the subject with the precision of a surgeon's scalpel. Do only the damage necessary to gain the information and no more. If the subject dies, you have failed."*

**—Dan Mitrione, the CIA's foremost authority on counterinsurgency torture techniques and Jim Jones's only childhood friend.**

James Warren Jones was born on May 13, 1931 to James T. and Lynetta Putnam Jones, poor itinerate farmers in the hamlet of Crete, Indiana. Lynetta was better educated than most men of her time. She had finished four years of college, but that had not taken the edge off this rough, argumentative, social outcast, who could swear like a drunken sailor and enjoyed rolling her own cigarettes that she puffed while passing the appalled local women. By most accounts, Jones's father was an uneducated, ill-mannered, bad-tempered loner, who worked part time as a laborer, but spent most of his time in bars, pool halls and the local Veteran's Administration Hospital. While serving in France during World War I, he had fallen victim to mustard gas and the slightest exertion left him breathless. Their small farm had been a gift from Lynetta's foster grandfather, but all that was lost during the Depression and the family moved five miles away to the nearest employment in Lynn, Indiana. Lynn offered the closest school system; a consideration as "Little Jim" approached school age.

Lynetta found a job and so did James T. who was appointed the "Night Marshal," a title that along with a gun, was bestowed upon him by the town fathers. At that time, in that place, the position of night marshal meant only one thing - head of the local chapter of the Ku Klux Klan's "wrecking crew." The KKK had a strong following in Indiana with over 300,000 members statewide, with most in small, rural communities like Lynn. Their national headquarters was only seventy miles away in Indianapolis, but most of their persecution of blacks took place in the countryside. Local KKK chapters would provide night time visits to other chapters' territories to carry out their dirty work, like burning black owned homes, cross burnings, and lynchings. That chapter would then reciprocate. In this way, Klan members were less likely to be identified, because their crimes were committed far from their home towns, while the local KKK members were certain to have a public alibi at the time. "Little Jim" was raised at the foot of his father, telling him stories about his raids on blacks the night before. It left a lasting impression.

Little Jim completed his first eleven years of education at the Washington Township School, where his teachers remembered him as a bright, but devilish, organizer with a foul mouth, no doubt inherited from his mother. Lynetta's influence was not all bad. She taught Little Jim the importance of reading. By the third grade, he was signing out library books intended for high school students. Even in grammar school, it was said that he was more knowledgeable than some of his teachers. Medicine, psychology, and Nazi Germany were his favorite subjects, and would guide him for the rest of his life.

Lynetta worked full-time at a local factory and "Big Jim" was no help at all with child care, so Little Jim was sent to a neighbor who babysat the child after school. It was Mrs. Myrtle Kennedy who first introduced Little Jim to religion. The Bible stories she read to him were interesting, but not as interesting as the power they exerted over her and her husband, who donated all their money and spare time to the local Methodist Church. Jones was not a joiner. He stood on the fringes of society and watched as if he was not a part of it and what he saw was a power that he wanted to command. He began touring various church services and became fascinated with the total control ministers and preachers exerted over their congregations. He was often seen at the home of a local Pentecostal minister, where he read from the Bible and practiced his oratory skills.

As sophisticated as Little Jim was, he was still only a child and so were his classmates, who he recruited for the "pretend church" that he conducted in the carriage house in his back yard. He officiated at services that were a combination science fair and religious revival. Jones sat in judgment in the only chair, while others gathered around the table to look into his microscope or marvel over the chicken to which he had attempted to graft a duck's leg. Sometimes he helped them with their homework. Sometimes he officiated at the funerals of their pets, some of which he probably killed just to be in charge.

A neighbor at the time would later recall his observations of Little Jim's pretend church. "He would preach a good sermon. I remember working about 200 feet from the Jones's place. He would have about ten youngsters in there, and he would put them through their paces, line them up, and make them march. He'd hit them with a stick and they'd scream and cry. I used to say, 'What's wrong with those other kids, putting up with it?', but they'd come back and play with him the next day. He had some kind of magnetism. I told my wife, "You know he's either going to do a lot of good or he's going to end up like Hitler."

"Heil Hitler!" **was** the password to get into Jones's pretend church. He often imitated his father by wearing a KKK white hood, but he was not savvy enough to wear it under the cover of night. He would parade through the neighborhood in full Klan apparel during the daylight.

Some time during this period, Big Jim's brother, Bill Jones, came to live with the family, but not for long. He died in a fall from the G Street bridge. His death was reported as a suicide, but many years later, Lynetta claimed to know that Uncle Bill was murdered. This was not the only time in young Jim's life that someone close to him died in a reported suicide that was really murder. It would happen again, at least five hundred times.

In Little Jim's junior year in high school, Big Jim and Lynetta separated and Lynetta moved young Jones closer to her new job in nearby Richmond, Indiana. Jones finished his senior year in Richmond, while working full-time as an orderly in a mental hospital where he met a nurse named Marceline Baldwin, the daughter of a prominent Republican city councilman. They were soon married. Marceline would stay by Jones's side until the bitter end in Jonestown, but not much has been written about her. Perhaps she was just overshadowed by Jones's extremely strong persona, but her voice was heard only a few times in the years to come. Once was in Los Angeles, when she ranted and raved to the police about the arrest of her husband on charges of lewd behavior, and once on the final tape recording of Jonestown when she pleaded with her husband not to kill the children in her care.

Some time around this period, Jones met Italian born, Indiana raised, Dan Mitrione. It was reported that they met in school, but Mitrione was about ten years Jones's senior. The two shared an interest in, of all things, torturing animals; something that was an outgrowth of Jones's earlier vivisection experiments. Mitrione would develop this macabre pastime into a lifelong career. Jones later recounted that growing up in Richmond, he knew, "A cruel, cruel person, even as a kid, a vicious racist—Dan Mitrione." Without credentials or a church, Jones decided to become a preacher to Richmond's poor black community. He would preach a good sermon on the street corner and convince his black audience to confess their sins and be forgiven. Many of their sins were crimes that Jones reported to Mitrione, who by then had been appointed the Richmond Police Department's juvenile officer. At the time, Richmond was suffering from a juvenile crime wave that was sweeping the city. Mitrione had promised the city fathers that he would clean it up, and he did, with help from his informant Jim Jones.

Over the next ten years, Jones studied business, law, and social services part-time at various colleges, finally receiving a bachelor's degree in education from Butler University. During this period, he continued preaching. He officially entered the ministry in 1952, when he accepted a position as student preacher at Somerset Methodist Church in a poor white neighborhood of Indianapolis. The church elders soon asked him to leave after he brought too many of his black street people into their conservative white congregation.

Meanwhile, Jones had established a name for himself at religious conventions in Columbus and Detroit. Even under the scrutiny of fellow preachers, Jones stole the show. He was a spell-binding orator with a particular talent to "discern"— a popular revivalist's trick. Jones would call out names of various people in the audience and "discern" some secret about them. He would disclose their phone or social security numbers or some ailment they suffered from. The subject would be asked to step forward and Jones would pray for them and, with a slap on the forehead, they would "fall out"— a phenomenon that is a combination of emotional overload and a sharp blow to the forehead. Some would rise immediately, brush themselves off, and return to their seats, while others would lie on the floor for hours, either quietly or in convulsions. This trick is not confined to revivalists. Even the Roman Catholic Church sanctions "falling out" practices though they are careful to use it sparingly. Immediately after the theatrics, the collection plate would be passed, followed by another subject being called forward and another collection plate. All the ministry know that discerning is a hoax, but they admired Jones's skill, his showmanship, and extraordinary memory, to say nothing about the very professional detective work required to gain the discerned information without the subject's knowledge. Jones could repeat social security, insurance policy, and driver's license numbers from dozens of people, all from memory. Never once in his career did he speak from notes. He performed fake cancer healings using rancid chicken livers and slight of hand. The "throat cancers" were performed on stage, but the anal cancers where performed back stage, leaving the details to the congregation's imagination. When he took his traveling circus on the road to Ohio, Jones would often use his aides as subjects. The advantage was they would not be recognized, but, the best discernings and healings were done on unsuspecting followers, who showed true amazement at the powers of this compelling young preacher.

After being kicked out of Somerset Methodist, Jones rented an abandoned church in a poor neighborhood of Indianapolis and started a business he called "Community Unity." The building was a church, but Community Unity was not. It was not recognized by any denomination. It was more of a social movement. Jones would conduct a Sunday service, but the real attraction lay in his ability to get as much public assistance to his followers as the law allowed. He helped his black followers fill out government forms to increase their financial support that he then required that they donate back to Community Unity.

Most of Jones's early followers were gleaned from other, targeted congregations. Jones would arrange to bring a contingent of his followers to another church service where he gave a guest sermon that far exceeded the skills of the resident minister. As was the custom, the next week, the targeted church would reciprocate and visit Jones's service. When the smoke cleared, many of the other congregation decided to convert to Jones's "church."

Jones wanted to portray his organization as multi-racial. He had Caucasian followers who blended into the group to give that impression, but upon closer observation, the whites were all administrative aides and the blacks were exclusively the sheep that Jones was fleecing. One early white recruit was a pharmaceutical company employee named Jack Beam—Jones's assistant pastor, bodyguard, and strong-arm man. Beam was the threat to keep followers in line, like the stick Jones had used on his grammar school-mates. All of Jones's finances came from the government. This included everything, right on up to the government surplus tractor that carried Congressman Ryan to his death. Jones purchased at auction a few former Indiana State Police patrol vehicles for Beam and others to use as company cars. The police required the official insignia to be removed, but Jones kept the familiar black and white color scheme that everyone recognized as a sign of authority and a threat to keep his black followers in line.

Jones sought out new black followers wherever and however he could. He even went door-to-door trying to recruit blacks by selling them monkeys. This deserves repeating. Yes, this fascist student of Nazi Germany sold monkeys door-to-door to recruit black followers that he ultimately intended to kill. Even at this early age, Jones would seem to have a sense of irony and his place in history. It was like he wanted someone in the future to look back on his life and say, "Oh, My God!" He would repeat this strange behavior dozens of times in the years to come.

Jones was extremely busy. He hosted three radio programs a week, all asking for donations. He conducted several services, each of which was intended to attract a different audience. There was the mainstream church service, the faith healing service, and the political service, in which he regaled against the communist influence and basically mirrored the McCarthy era witch hunt. He rarely mentioned God and was more likely to quote newspaper articles than the Bible. His was a down-to-earth ministry, more concerned with pleasing the government for more public assistance than pleasing God for some afterlife reward.

Jones established Jim/Lu/Mar; an Indiana for profit corporation, named after himself, his mother, and his wife, whose stated purpose was to "receive donations of real estate." Like his "Wings of Deliverance" established later, despite the fact that they were licensed "profit-making" businesses, Jones filed only one tax return for Wings of Deliverance and no others, yet he was never in trouble with the IRS, enjoying a certain protection. To the government, Jones's activities were "hands off".

Jones proceeded to target elderly black people who owned their homes. He promised to take care of them for the rest of their lives if they willed their property to Jim/Lu/Mar, and many did. Proprietary homes like this were common, but unfortunately for the residents, there was nothing common about Jim Jones. He established several elderly care facilities, one in his own home. He hired Mable Stewart as his nursing home supervisor. On one trip to recruit followers in Hamilton, Ohio, Jones insisted that Mable and her staff of four ride in one car, along with Stephanie, his wife's cousin, who had come to live with the Joneses. On the way home, Mable, her staff, and Stephanie were killed in a car crash. The car had been sabotaged and, at first, the police suspected that it was done by Jones, but they dismissed this theory because his young niece was among the victims. In truth, Jones was silencing Mable and her staff, who were raising objections about the untimely deaths of several of the elderly residents in their care. Once his followers willed their properties to Jones, their life expectancy was severely shortened. It was a technique he repeated throughout his career.

Jones hit upon a way to help the federal government remedy a problem they had, while at the same time, help himself. The South Korean government was petitioning the US to take responsibility for the orphans fathered by US troops during the Korean War. These racially-mixed rejects of Korean society were being housed in special orphanages in Seoul because racial prejudices in Korea were extreme, even by American standards. Jones encouraged his congregation to adopt these children and set the example by adopting two— two year old Lew Eric and a four-year-old girl he renamed Stephanie after his wife's deceased cousin. With the addition of a young black boy, the first ever to be adopted by a Caucasian family in Indiana, and a blue-eyed blonde, Jones assembled his "Rainbow Family," as he called them, that helped him present the public persona of a multi-racial socialist to disguise the fact that he was really a racist.

By 1956, Jones had amassed enough money to purchase a modest church in the Indianapolis inner-city that he named "Wings of Deliverance." Soon after, Jones organized a huge five-day, religious convention in a rented hall in Indianapolis. Upwards of 11,000 people attended the opening ceremonies. There were several speakers, but, as usual, Jones stole the show. Jones made so much money from the convention that within the year, he purchased a second, more impressive, building from Rabbi Maurice Davis and renamed his group, "The People's Temple Full Gospel Church." Jones would go on to purchase two other houses of worship, one in San Francisco and one in Los Angeles. Against all odds, all three were former Jewish synagogues. Jones preferred the buildings that looked like houses of worship but without the entrapments of Christianity. There were no crosses or stained glass images of saints. He liked the eternal flame and kept it lit for services. It could not escape this student of Nazi Germany that the Nazis had built the Auschwitz Concentration Camp on land they had confiscated from Jewish farmers.

By 1960, the Peoples Temple social programs exceeded those offered by the City of Indianapolis. Their soup kitchens fed over a hundred people a day. They operated youth centers to educate and entertain idle teenagers and several nursing care facilities for the elderly; at least those who had property or a pension to donate to the cause. These programs were good publicity, but they were also profitable. Jones gave only $25 a week to the soup kitchens. Most of the food came from grocery stores and restaurants that gladly gave the Peoples Temple their over-ripened, expired food in exchange for inflated tax deductions. Some of the food ended up in the soup kitchen, but only after the seniors in his charge had their fill. Jones's "good work" caught the attention of the Disciples of Christ, that sanctioned him and his Peoples Temple as one of their own, a tax-exempt status he enjoyed until the very end in Jonestown. For his efforts, Jones was appointed Director of Indianapolis's Human Rights Commission.

Jones recognized that nothing could galvanize and strengthen a group more than the threat of a perceived common enemy. Since none existed, he created one. His followers began receiving, late night, threatening phone calls from the "American Nazi Party" or the "Ku Klux Klan," Arriving at Sunday services, they found their pets dead on the steps, their throats slit and the blood running down into the street. The building had been vandalized the night before. Black spray paint spelled out, "Nigger Lover" and there were swastikas painted everywhere. Jones took the podium and after an uncomfortably long silence (as was Hitler's style), he screamed, "Nigger lover! Nigger lover! You better believe I'm a nigger lover!" The congregation erupted into wild cheers and applause. It was one of his largest collection plates ever. It was remarkable what Jones could do with just a dollar can of spray paint and a knife.

Meanwhile, Jones's good friend, Dan Mitrione, had been appointed Richmond's Chief of Police. Soon after, he joined the FBI and soon after that, in 1960, he joined the CIA as their expert in severe interrogation, in other words, torture. At first, the CIA set up shop in Mitrione's basement that had been soundproofed so the neighbors could not hear the screams of his victims. South American intelligence, military and police officials were brought in for Mitrione's one day seminar on how to extract information from uncooperative subjects. In the morning session, Mitrione lectured on psychology and the human nervous system. In the afternoon, a homeless person was kidnapped off the street, stripped naked and restrained. Mitrione attached electrodes to their genitals and shocked them repeatedly, slowly increasing the intensity and duration. The object was to reach that level where the subject abandoned his innermost beliefs. Once attained, he would tell the interrogator anything he wanted to know. Mitrione warned his students, "If the subject dies, you have failed."

After class, the homeless person was killed, redressed and, dumped back on the street. The risk of killing Americans on American soil did not escape the CIA, who were well aware that it was illegal for them to even operate in the United States. So, they decided that Mitrione should travel to South America and set up his torture school anywhere but on US soil. In late 1960 or early 1961, the US State Department's International Cooperation Administration sent Mitrione to Brazil to "teach advanced counterinsurgency techniques" to their police and military. Before he left, Mitrione recruited his old friend, Jim Jones, to join the CIA.

Jones entered the CIA on the shirttails of Dan Mitrione, but with good reason— he had much to offer the Company. It is true that Jones was a sociopath, but he was a very talented sociopath. He had a knowledge of human psychology that rivaled the professionals, but without the restrictions of the Hippocratic Oath. Years later, attorney Charles Garry described him as having more charisma than anyone he had ever met. Jones's aura was so strong, so compelling, that his surviving followers recounted that it was impossible for them to even think for themselves when he was in the room. Whether this was a God-given talent or acquired from years of studying techniques of mind control, whether he used hypnosis or some unknown form of coercion, the bottom line was **Jim Jones could convince anyone to do anything.** Ultimately, the CIA would test his skills in Jonestown.

Jones's first foreign assignments with the CIA required him to be away from Indianapolis for two or three years and he only had two or three weeks to arrange for someone to take care of his little empire in his absence. His in-laws, the Baldwins, agreed to manage his nursing home businesses, but that left the Peoples Temple. His new employers came to his aid when they introduced him to Ed Malmin, a Chicago street thug, turned preacher, who had worked for the Company in Brazil. It was commonplace for the CIA to use missionaries as operatives or claim that operatives were missionaries. Malmin's case was probably the later. After Jonestown, the practice of using missionary spies was outlawed by Congress, but it was standard procedure in the early 1960s. Malmin's daughter had grown up in Brazil and was fluent in both English and Portuguese. So it was decided that Ed Malmin would mind Jones's Indianapolis church in his absence while his daughter, Bonnie, would be Jones's interpreter in Brazil. Jones told his followers that he was leaving to do missionary work in South America. They were disappointed, but had no choice but to accept it.

Jones called it, "The Big Time," but not even his closest aides knew what he meant. First he had to go to a CIA camp for indoctrination. Jones and his wife flew to Hawaii for "a two week vacation" that was really spent in spy school at a US Naval Base. They then flew to Georgetown, British Guiana in South America, where Jones dove head long into a political struggle of continental proportions. Without free slave labor, the British government could no longer make a profit from British Guiana. They were willing to grant their colony independence, but they still wanted to maintain control. However, the upcoming elections did not look favorable for British or US interests. Two opposing ethnic factions were fighting for power. First, there were the descendants of the black slaves that British businessmen had imported to work in their sugar cane fields. This group was represented by Linden 'Forbes' Burnham, who by all accounts was a puppet of the British and the CIA. Burnham had been vetted by the British while studying law at the University of London, after which he traveled to the US were the CIA added their blessing. The second group were descendants of East Indian indentured servants, also imported to work in the sugar cane fields. This group was headed by Cheddi Jagan, an avowed communist, and it looked like Jagan was going to win the election. The CIA would not tolerate another communist country in the Western Hemisphere. They fought with everything they had, including their asset Jim Jones.

Jones worked under Richard Welch, the US ambassador to Guiana, and together they devised a plan to destroy Cheddi Jagan's career. With Jones's powers of persuasion and a pocket full of cash, he recruited poor black street people to disrupt Jagan's campaign. They ransacked Jagan's headquarters, threatened his supporters, and almost totally destroyed the economy of the entire country. That, along with Jones's manipulation of election results was enough to eventually get Forbes Burnham elected Premier and later Prime Minister. Jones's work, in what was now called Guyana, was finished and he flew to Belo Horizonte, Brazil to join his old friend Dan Mitrione.

Jones moved into 203 Rua Maraba, a luxurious home the CIA had rented for him in an upper class neighborhood close to Mitrione. Bonnie Malmin soon moved in. Jones tried to continue with his initial cover as a missionary, but aside from carrying a Bible, his lifestyle did not reflect that story. He was provided with a live-in maid and cook who were confined to the property out of fear they might be questioned in public. There were Brazilian military in and out of Jones's house at all hours of the day and night. US Embassy personnel were daily visitors, often delivering groceries, and Jones's neighbors became suspicious. He told some that he was working for the Eureka commercial laundry, but no one believed him. Jones had a different cover story for each of his neighbors. To one, he was a "missionary," to another he was a "traffic advisor," to another, he was "a retired US navy officer," to another, he was "Naval Intelligence," Either he could not keep his story straight or he was deliberately confusing his suspicious neighbors. One neighbor woman called him, "Just a gangster with a Bible."

What Jones was really doing was recruiting Brazilian military and ex-military personnel to work as mercenaries in a war that was an ocean away in the South African country of Angola. Angola's war of Independence started that same year and the US had an interest not in securing Angola's independence from Portugal, but in who would rule the country afterwards. 1961 was a very volatile year. It was the height of the Cold War and the Cuban missile crisis. The Soviets and Cubans were moving tens of thousands of troops into Angola, in order to create another communist country in the aftermath of what promised to be a successful war of independence from Portugal. The US had a vested interest in stopping the communists, but did not want to use US troops that could trigger a nuclear holocaust in South Africa. What they really coveted was Angola's vast off-shore oil reserves. The CIA decided to fight a once removed war with mercenaries, but that presented a problem. Angolans are blacks who speak Portuguese. There is only one other place in the world where that combination can be found, and that is in Brazil.

Jones's neighbors directly across the street were two lawyers, Marco and Elza Rocha. Elza sometimes translated legal documents for Jones, while Marco kept surveillance on his activities. Marco was working for a local police detective who suspected that Jones was CIA. There were good reasons why this was important to the Brazilian government because, along with his other assignments, Jones was recruiting Brazilian military for another CIA project, he was planning a military coup that would bring down the Brazilian government just two years later.

Bonnie Malmin was an extremely attractive sixteen-year-old, fair skinned, buxom blonde and the perfect lure for young Brazilian soldiers. Bonnie's beauty and Jones's masterful ability to recruit blacks were a tremendous success. They signed up thousands of recruits. Some were put on the CIA's payroll immediately and sent to Angola. Most were held in reserve for what the CIA knew would be an internal power struggle after the war of independence was won. The project was run by Admiral Charles Buford, who Jones worked for. Later Buford's daughter Terri, worked for Jones as his most trusted aide in Jonestown.

Jones and Malmin did a stellar job in Belo Horizonte, with everything except their own cover. The death blow came in a local newspaper feature article about Jones that described him as "that flamboyant American who claims to be a missionary, but who we all know is CIA." Bonnie reportedly attempted suicide, but was rescued and sent back to the states. Mission accomplished, translator gone, cover blown, Jones left Belo Horizonte for a one-year stay in a luxurious high-rise apartment overlooking the exclusive Cop Cabaña Beach in Rio de Janeiro, but not before the police detective who was investigating him died unexpectedly just before he finished his final report. Dan Mitrione soon followed Jones to Rio.

It was some time during this period that Jones pressured the Company for a face-to-face meeting with Josep Mengele who the CIA was harboring in Brazil. They agreed because Mengele could be of value to Jones in his next assignment, consolidating the results of their **MK ULTRA** experiments into comprehensive weapons of mind control that had been initiated by Nazi Paperclip scientists.

**MK ULTRA** was a series of 160 separate experiments, conducted by or under the CIA in universities, research faculties, mental hospitals, military bases, and prisons throughout the United States and Canada that begun in 1953. Unwitting human subjects were subjected to various experiments designed to alter brain functions and mental states through the use of torture, drugs, hypnosis, sensory deprivation, sexual, and verbal abuse. Originally, it was intended as a study in interrogating uncooperative wartime prisoners, but it soon expanded to include studies in the Noetic sciences, like telekinesis, astral projection, remote viewing, memory erasure, intention and the creation of multiple personalities designed to produce assassins, as fictionalized in books and movies such as "The Manchurian Candidate," and "The Bourne Identity." The Soviets, the Chinese and the North Koreans had similar programs and the US needed to keep pace. One-sixth of the CIA's budget was allocated to **MK ULTRA**. The Army, Navy and Air Force all played a role with many of our enlisted men being used as guinea pigs.

"MK" designated that the project was sponsored by the CIA's Technical Services Staff though some claim that it is the German abbreviation of "Mind Control." "ULTRA" designated the most top secret classification in World War II intelligence. The project had its origins in Operation Paperclip. Nazi scientists brought into the CIA had made tremendous strides in interrogation techniques using torture, brainwashing, and other forms of coercion, and the CIA wanted to embellish on their findings. This was a twenty-five year program, that cost over $25 million dollars. It had other names: **MK ARTICHOKE, MK BLUEBIRD, MK NAOMI, MK SEARCH** and **STARGATE,** but all of them fell under the umbrella of **MK ULTRA.**

Some of the experimentation had to do with mind altering drugs, like LSD and mescaline and were conducted by the army in the early 1950s. LSD was actually invented by a CIA doctor as a truth serum for interrogating Soviet agents. Though never published, it is difficult to accept that this effort did not include the army's Director of Chemical and Biological Warfare, who, at the time was Dr. Lawrence Layton and whose wife had strong ties to Operation Paperclip. Torture was another subject and the CIA's expert on torture was Dan Mitrione. With the Laytons on one side and Mitrione on the other, Jim Jones was right in the middle.

Many of these experiments were conducted in the 1950s and ten years later, no one had ever reviewed the results. This was the early 1960s and not even the CIA was computerized. The files were all on paper, hundreds of thousands of pages, most of which were just raw data that had never been read, more or less compiled. Jones had about ten years to review and copy the files before CIA Director Richard Helmes succumbed to congressional pressure and ordered them destroyed in 1973 as Jones embarked on the ultimate **MK ULTRA** project known as Jonestown.

While supposedly in Rio, Jones may have traveled to other countries, but this cannot be confirmed. What can be confirmed is that he had left the US with two passports; #0111788 and #22898751. For the rest of his public career, he was very proud of the photo he displayed in his office of himself, his wife, and a man who looked remarkably like Fidel Castro. Since Castro never left Cuba, Jones must have traveled there.

Allow me to digress for a moment. Castro is not who we are duped into believing he is. Concentrate on reality, not rhetoric. The CIA trained Castro as an actor in Hollywood. He even appeared as an extra in a few movies. We sent him back to Cuba to overthrow Baptista, after which he visited Washington D.C. to meet with then Vice President Richard Nixon for a top secret strategy session. After their meeting, in April of 1959, Nixon sent a confidential memorandum to the CIA, the State Department, and the White House that claimed Castro was a communist and should be treated accordingly. It was not Castro who told the world that he was a communist, it was "Tricky Dick" Nixon. Castro then proceeded to "supposedly" turned on us. What he really did was give the US access to Soviet military technology. In exchange, we gathered up all his militant enemies and sent them into a suicide mission called the Bay of Pigs Invasion. The CIA then circulated wild, inflammatory rumors that they wanted to kill Castro with Thallium salts to make his beard fall out or poison pens or exploding cigars. Castro often appeared in public. A simple sniper shot to the head would have sufficed. The CIA did not want to kill Castro. Castro was their man. The Soviets wanted a foothold in the Western Hemisphere and the CIA handed them Cuba on a silver platter.

In the year that Jones spent in Rio, he was very busy with a few assignments. First, there were the **MK ULTRA** files to review. There were boxes and boxes of experiment data that needed to be analyzed and condensed into some sort of comprehensive overview. He also continued meeting with Mengele and accepted a position as an investment salesman with Invesco, S.A. His job never provided any income for Jones. He was "commission only," and during his three-month stay with the firm, he never sold anything. What his involvement really provided was an introduction into the Nazi underground. One of Invesco's founders had been a Nazi spy. Invesco was established as the last stop on the "Rat Run" to help launder and liquidate assets of hundreds of Nazis who had fled to Brazil after World War II. Invesco pioneered the sale of mutual funds in South America and provided a conduit to launder Nazi wealth, much of which was in stolen art works. The Nazis had stolen over 20% of Europe's art. What little was later recovered was proven to be masterful forgeries. The Nazis kept the originals and needed to liquidate them. Invesco had associates in a loose-knit organization of art galleries. There were also allegations that they were involved in heroin smuggling, which will come into play later in this story. By 1967, Invesco had fulfilled its purpose and closed its operation.

As early as 1962, at least a rough outline of the ultimate **MK ULTRA** experiments had been written. They needed a quantitative representation of the targeted population. Various cocktails of promising psychotropic drugs would be administered. The dosage had to be sufficient to totally destroy the subject's will, but not so strong as to impede their ability to work or be detected in routine medical examinations. And what was the ultimate test of whether they were under total control? There was only one. Jim Jones would ask them to kill themselves.

# F O U R

## THE BIG TIME

*"Ninety-five percent of humanity produces nothing but excrement."*

**—Leonardo Da Vinci.**

The following chapter is based on historical facts, but artistic license was used to recreate the private conversation between Jim Jones and Josef Mengele in order for the reader to get a better understanding of the first Holocaust as a prerequisite to understanding the second.

Dr. Josep Mengele was the most wanted, the most dangerous, and the most valuable man in the world. "The Angel of Death" had information that could alter history. To keep him from falling into Soviet hands, the CIA brought him into Operation Paperclip, but he was far too volatile to house in the United States, so they hid him in South America where he continued to study the blood samples he had taken from Auschwitz.

It was 1962, and Jim Jones was lost in a maze of confusing, winding mountain roads in Brazil. Finally, he found the remote farm in Serra Negro that Mengele managed. A laborer met him at the gate and motioned for him to follow. He was led to a fruit tree orchard and a group of workers surrounding a man, who was pointing out branches for them to prune. The man wore a large hat, that Jones later learned he always wore, to conceal his prominent forehead that he feared might give away his true identity, but Jones knew it was Mengele the instant he opened his mouth to expose the gap between his two front teeth that was wide enough to insert a wooden match stick. Mengele concentrated on his work, continuing to point out branches, while talking to Jones as if he was not even there.

"We cut this one because it is infected with gall, a fatal fungus that will spread to the rest of the tree and the entire orchard if it isn't removed and burned. This one we cut to open the tree's interior to allow better air circulation and sunlight to increase productivity. These two branches are crossing and rubbing against each other. Both will die unless we remove the weaker one. There are many reasons to eliminate a branch to benefit the orchard.

How much more important is it to eliminate 'useless eaters' to benefit mankind?"

Mengele motioned Jones to follow him to a small concrete out building near the farmhouse. Inside the stucco-clad room was a rustic table and two chairs. On the table was a pitcher of milk, a bowl of fruit, and a candle. A single window overlooked the orchard. They sat down.

"Are you comfortable?" asked Mengele and Jones replied, "Yes, sir."

Mengele stood, walked over to the door, locked it with a skeleton key, threw the key out the open window, closed the wooden window shutters, and padlocked them, lit the candle and returning to his chair.

"Are you still comfortable?" he asked.

"Uh, yes, sir, Jones responded, out of deference to his host, but it was not true. He felt uneasy.

"We only have enough food to survive for a few days. Are you still comfortable?" This time, Jones did not answer.

"Suppose we were not alone. Suppose there were twenty additional people locked in this room with us. Would you still feel comfortable?

"No!", Jones quickly responded. "There's not enough food or room or air. We would all die very quickly."

"Exactly, but what you fail to understand is that this locked room is the planet Earth. What you would do to survive in this room is what you need to do to survive on this planet. What would you do?"

"I'd have to eliminate most of them, just to survive another day."

"Which ones?" Mengele asked.

"The ones who took more than their share of the food or rather, the ones who took more than they added to the group."

Mengele poured a glass of milk and sat back in his chair, obviously deep in thought.

"There are only two gifted people in this world; Germans and Jews, and it's a question of who will be superior. Germans will succeed. Our plan is to purify the human race in 120 years. We are already twenty years into that schedule, but we can't finish it alone. One hundred and twenty years represents the productive lives of three or four generations. There comes a time to pass the torch to younger blood and we have chosen you. We have followed your career for some time now and believe that you are the one."

Jones was shocked. He had hoped that Mengele might just give him some advice about his work or reveal some Nazi secret he could bring back to his CIA sponsors. He never expected anything even remotely like this.

"You will need to make sacrifices, but there will be rewards as well. Are you willing to take up the task that we started?"

"Yes, but the Jews are so sensitive to anything like this, they'll stop me immediately."

Mengele laughed out loud, showing the gap between his teeth. "The Jews will be your greatest ally. Those self-pitying martyrs have convinced the world that the Holocaust was anti-Semitic and intended solely to persecute them. The truth is they were the last to be eliminated; almost an afterthought. Many survived to tell their 'poor me' stories and show their tattoos to the camera. Tell me, how did we identify Jews in the ghettos?"

"With a yellow star of David sewn to their outer clothing", Jones responded.

"Exactly, but did you know that badge was only one of thirty-eight such primary badges? Faggots wore pink triangles. We burned over 250,000 faggots in just two years, more than they did in every town square in Europe during the entire Middle Ages. The badge for a drug addict was a hypodermic needle. And then there were an infinite number of combination badges. A homosexual drug addict wore a pink triangle with a hypodermic needle through it. The list was endless, but we managed to send all of them to the gas chambers very early on before we even considered the Jewish question. No one survived these first groups to cry 'poor me'. First, we eliminated the 'Life Unworthy of Life'. These were the retarded, the insane, the criminal or genetically defective parasites that didn't contribute to society. Then there were the Roma or 'Gypsies' as you call them, Jehovah Witnesses, communists, Slavs, intellectuals, academics, alcoholics, niggers, swing dancers and political opponents. Did you know we guillotined over 20,000 political critics in public executions? We chopped off more heads than they did in the entire French Revolution. All of these groups were eliminated, but you will never hear anyone lamenting their fate because, unlike the Jews, we left no survivors to testify.

"Niggers in pre-war Germany? Alcoholics? Swing dancers?" Jones was obviously confused.

"Yes, niggers in Germany, but we didn't exactly kill them, we destroyed their lineage. There is a region between Germany and France called Alsace Lorraine that has changed hands for hundreds of years depending on who won the previous war. At the end of World War I, it was ceded to France who brought in French Foreign legion troops from North Africa to guard the border. By the time we regained the territory, these nigger soldiers had interbred with the local German women and had to be stopped before they further polluted the gene pool. Luckily, they were all about the same age and so were their mulatto offspring. Their wives had grown too old to have additional children so we just sterilized their children and stopped the nigger blood from tainting the pure Arian race. We did this quietly, without even telling the parents so as not to offend the German mothers. Alcoholism is a genetic disorder, passed from one generation to the next. Eliminate all alcoholics and there is a good chance of breaking the chain and eliminating the condition forever. We saw swing dancers as a negative Nigger influence on civilized society. We knew it would evolve into promiscuous sex, drugs, debauchery, and a general decay of the social structure. We raided their night clubs, arrested them all, and sent them to work and die in concentration camp factories. Judging from what has happened in the world since, we were right, but we failed to complete the task. There is a lot of work that remains and only 100 years to complete it. Do your part, contribute, stay on schedule. Do whatever the CIA asks of you, but work under their protection to accomplish our agenda."

Mengele fell silent, just staring at the wall. "They are going to kill me, maybe even you, but we can't let fear deter us. It is our duty to secure the success of the human race. No one else is willing to do what's necessary."

With that, Mengele rose, went to the door, and knocked four times. A farm worker unlocked the door and escorted Jones to the front gate ending the first of many such meetings he would have with the 'Angel of Death' over the next year. As he walked to his car, Jones's mind was racing with endless future possibilities, but above all else he felt a sense of euphoria that finally, his father would have been proud.

# F I V E

## CALIFORNIA OR BUST

*"It is best to avoid the beginnings of evil...there are a thousand hacking at the branches of evil to one who is striking at the root."*

**—Henry David Thoreau.**

At this point in time, Jim Jones did not have much money. Born into poverty, he had a few low paying jobs and most of those were part-time. His fledgling ministry was as much of a financial drain as it was a profit making business. So how could he afford his lifestyle? He just returned from a two-week "vacation" in Hawaii, six months in British Guiana, six months in an upscale rented house in Belo Horizonte followed by a year in a luxury apartment on the Cop Cabaña Beach in Rio. How did he pay for all of this? The answer is simple; he did not. The CIA paid his bills. Jones returned to the US in 1963 with $100,000 in seed money that was allegedly given to him by the wife of the US ambassador to Brazil but, from this point forward, financially, he had to fend for himself.

Jones returned to Indianapolis and Mengele went back to the small, rural community of Candido Godai, Brazil to continue his study of twins. Candido Godai had been founded by German immigrants in the early 1900's and had an international reputation for producing twins. More than four times the rate of any other place on earth. The residents remember the German doctor who visited them on occasion to give the young woman "vitamin" shots. Some have suggested that the twin phenomenon was a natural result of only twelve German families, having settled the town and one or more having a genetic predisposition to produce twins. Whether Mengele was there to study an anomaly that existed in nature or to use the community as a laboratory to create twins, may never be known. In any event, the clock was ticking on the Nazi's 120-year goal to purify the human race.

Mitrione remained behind in Brazil to oversee the military coup that successfully toppled the government a few months later.

Jones settled back into Indianapolis and spent his time studying the intricacies of the federal government and how taxpayers' money was spent. It was Jones's mastery of government finances that allowed him to use government programs to fund his Peoples Temple and the ensuing experiments. He gathered together a core group of aides who were mostly wealthy, intelligent, well-educated, Caucasian young women. Some came from families with ties to the intelligence community, but most were just worker bees who did what they were told out of loyalty to Jones and never really understood the results of their efforts. Jones organized several departments. One was the "Planning Commission," the ruling class of his organization, comprised of his closest aides, but the most interesting was the "Department of Diversions," that was charged with covert operations. Jones employed them as spies to create extensive files on his followers and anyone else who came into contact with him. They would rifle through a subject's garbage looking for personal correspondence, bills, or anything that might add to their knowledge of the targeted person. Two agents, posing as a married couple, would knock on a subject's door, claim their car had broken down, and ask to use the phone. While one phoned, the other would ask to use the bathroom and, while inside, make copious notes on the contents of the medicine cabinet. Hospitals, doctors, and prescriptions were all noted. Jones would send his "Department of Diversion" agents on recon missions armed only with a dog leash. If caught snooping around a neighborhood, they could always say they were looking for a lost dog. Sometimes, they even wore wigs and blackface in order to blend into the black neighborhoods under surveillance. Their intelligence gathering techniques rivaled those of the CIA, because whether they realized it or not, they were the CIA.

Jones used the data in his services to reveal private information about a parishioner who would be astounded and convinced of his divine powers. It was intended to create the first page in their file—a blank piece of paper that Jones had the subject sign at the bottom as a test of their loyalty. He would later type in confessions to horrific crimes to blackmail the subject into transferring their money, possessions, and real estate..

**The Peoples Temple was not a religion.** This can not be emphasized enough. **The Peoples Temple was not a religion.** It did have all the entrapments of a religion, but it was more of a social movement. There was a "church," a pulpit, a minister in robes, a choir, and fake faith healings, but that was the extent of it. Jones never studied to be a minister. His credentials were mail order or honorary, based only upon his desire to be addressed as "father," as he required of his followers. God was never mentioned except when Jones called him the "Impotent Sky God," powerless to affect anything in this world. Jones would spit on the Bible, stomp on it, kick it into the congregation, talk about using its pages as toilet paper, and then stand as living proof that the "Impotent Sky God" was powerless to retaliate. There was no God in heaven, there was only Jim Jones on Earth and he was God.

In 1965, he moved his church to Mendocino County, California, but he did not take everyone. He selected about eighty individuals, based on their dossiers, and left the rest behind, a practice he repeated years later when he moved only 1,200 of his 5,000 followers to Guyana. There are at least four possible reasons why Jones moved to Mendocino. First, the stated reason, that he was responding to an article in **Esquire Magazine** that identified Ukiah, California as one of the nine safest places to hide in the event of a nuclear war. Taking into account proximity to military targets, prevailing winds, and sustainable food supplies, the article attempted to identify the nine places in the world to survive a nuclear holocaust. The article was written almost tongue-in-cheek, therefore difficult to accept that Jones had been taken in by it, but it could possibly have been a coded message. One of the nine places was Belo Horizonte, Brazil that Jones had just left, prior to the article's publication. Another was Guadalajara, Mexico where he eventually sent one of his followers to medical school— the one who ultimately mixed the poison in Jonestown. The next reason was the Mendocino State Mental Hospital. Jones sent the children of his followers to Santa Rosa Junior College to earn degrees in nursing and then strategically placed them in the hospital. His army of seventy nurses would be the backbone of his medical staff and their work at the hospital to "de-institutionalize" the patients, altered the entire US government's treatment of the mentally ill.

Another reason may have been Mendocino County's reputation as the nation's premier producer of high-quality marijuana, the largest agricultural cash crop in California. Law enforcement officials in South America suspected that Jones was brokering drugs between Bolivia, Brazil, Guyana, and the US. Jones never touched the drugs, only provided the money and the contacts to turn $100,000 of legal coca leaves in Bolivia into $100 million dollars of illegal cocaine in the US. Jones would eventually control the entire county and presumably the marijuana crop. He may have lost touch with his South American suppliers, but not his US customers. This is not the only time that the CIA has been accused of profiting from the drug trade to finance their covert operations. Drugs may have been the reason he moved to Mendocino. Lastly, Jones needed black subjects for his experiments and there were few in Indiana where the rule was "Nigger don't let the the sun set on you here." A pool of a least 5,000 black and/or homosexual followers were needed in order for him to select the perfect 1,200 "test persons" for his experiments. Nearby San Francisco provided just such a pool.

A year earlier, California succumbed to public pressure and stopped the forced sterilization of black welfare recipients, felons, parolees, and prisoners. As late as 1964, even progressive California looked a lot like Nazi Germany.

Jones moved his selected congregation to Ukiah, California (Redwood Valley to be exact). He purchased a forty-acre ranch that he sarcastically named, "Happy Acres." He immediately set out to attack the Mendocino County infrastructure with a vengeance. Mendocino was a sparsely populated rural county. It was small enough for Jones to control, remote enough to hide his activities, and close enough to his ultimate destination- San Francisco. His first concern was housing his followers. He purchased a motel, an apartment house, a rest home, and several single family houses. Since a "family" is anyone willing to live communally, he packed as many people into the houses as the structures could hold. He somehow managed to be appointed foreman of the Mendocino County Grand Jury. Basically, he was the king of the county able to bring charges against or protect anyone he so chose. His first paying job was teaching American History and Government in the county's adult education program. His classes were closed to everyone but his aides, which allowed him to advance his agenda with government support. In 1967, he formed the Legal Services Foundation of Mendocino County to offer free legal advice to the county's poor, but what he really did was identify vulnerable candidates for his Peoples Temple. In 1968, he was appointed to the Juvenile Justice Commission, another rich source of recruits.

The Peoples Temple met in a number of rented places during this period, first in the Evangelical Free Church until they kicked them out, then in a 4-H exhibition barn at the Mendocino County Fairgrounds, until they kicked them out and left Jones with nowhere to hold services but his garage. With his back to the wall, he decided to build his "church" at his residence. It took three building permits to construct his "church" built around an enclosed swimming pool.

Jones's compound looked like a concentration camp. It was surrounded by chain link fences, barbed wire, guard towers, and uniformed military personnel armed with automatic weapons. Attack dogs patrolled the perimeter. It looked like a concentration camp because it was. The neighbors complained to the authorities, but nothing was done, because, by then Jones controlled the county.

The families that Jones brought from Indianapolis included many young girls, who would grow into young woman, who Jones found easier to control and placed in important positions in the county's welfare departments. Eventually, most of the county's foster children and anyone else with government support were brought under Jones's control. He received the money and doled out their support in communal homes that were supported by additional government programs. In Mendocino, it was impossible to receive public assistance without first joining the Peoples Temple. Social Security and disability recipients, children in foster care, welfare recipients, all had to join or they would lose their support. Such was the strangle-hold that Jones had on Mendocino County's poor.

Tim Stoen joined the Peoples Temple some time during this period. He was a young flashy California lawyer, a bachelor who drove a Porsche. Stoen was CIA, or at least the East Germans thought so. In the early 1960s, while Jones was working in South America, Stoen was arrested in East Germany for espionage when he was caught photographing sensitive Soviet military instillations. He was held for nine days, but a deal was struck and he was released. Stoen was Mendocino County's Assistant District Attorney, well placed to help the county's foreman of the Grand Jury: his client, pastor, and friend, Jim Jones.

Jim Jones had absolutely no regard for the law, but he was so clever that most of his criminal activities went undetected. On rare occasions, he did have run-ins with the authorities and he always turned to Tim Stoen, who never failed to rescue him. A good example was the "Powered Milk Incident."

Jones confiscated all of his follower's government support money, but he still needed to feed them. The US Department of Agriculture distributed powdered milk to the poor through a program that was exclusively administered in Mendocino County by a woman named Eunice Mock. On March 5, 1971, Ms. Mock and a colleague were driving on a back road in Mendocino when they observed two open pick-up trucks with upwards of eighty cases of clearly marked USDA powdered milk. She had no knowledge of such a large shipment and proceeded to follow them. Temple member James Bogue realized he was being followed and pulled over to confront Ms. Mock. He tried to intimidate her by shouting that the milk was for poor people and none of her business. She wrote down the license plate numbers and filed a complaint with the Department of Agriculture, that dispatched two investigators to

40

Jones's home, because the plates were registered to the Peoples Temple. Jones denied any knowledge of the powdered milk or the trucks. He grabbed his chest, feigning a heart attack, and retired to his bedroom where he called Tim Stoen. Stoen appeared on the scene to defend Jones, the Peoples Temple and Bogue but the investigators were not satisfied. Stoen then called San Francisco City Supervisor Dianne Finestein to stop the investigation because the powdered milk had originated in San Francisco from the Community Health Alliance, headed by Peter Holmes, a Peoples Temple member Jones had placed in that position, possibly with help from Dr. Layton who, at the time, was the Director of the USDA's Western Regional Laboratory. Holmes was clearly stealing government food for Jones. The investigation continued for several weeks. Eventually, Jones returned the powdered milk to the San Francisco warehouse, but   Peter Holmes was forced to resign. No charges were ever filed.

Jones purchased a small shopping mall in Redwood Valley and proceeded to open several businesses. Two of these were thrift stores where temple followers were forced to donate their time and valuables. Living communally, they no longer needed their own furniture, kitchen utensils, surplus clothing, or any other possessions.  In addition to the money that thrift stores provided to the temple coffers, they also made it very difficult for the parishioners to quit the temple and return to their previous lives, because those lives had been sold and no longer existed. Jones also opened Mendocino's only telephone answering service. In a time before answering machines, this reasonably priced service allowed Jones to monitor the communications of the many local residents, who unknowingly subscribed to what was basically a phone tap.

The temple's money was piling up so fast that Stoen warned Jones that it would draw unwanted legal attention and advised him to spread it out evenly among no less than fifteen different banks.

Many local residents speculated that the main reason Jones moved to Mendocino was the Mendocino State Mental Hospital. Jones would use the daughters of his core group of followers in a long term plan to build a medical staff for his ultimate experiments in Jonestown. He sent each to the Santa Rosa Junior College were they received degrees in nursing and medical records keeping and then on to work at the State Mental Hospital. Slowly, one at a time, Jones convinced the authorities, many of whom were his own followers, that the hospital's patients were not a threat to themselves or society and should be released to live normal lives under his care. Jones took the patients and their support checks under his wing, which pleased the State of California because paying the Peoples Temple cost less than operating the hospital. Eventually, all the patients were released to Jones and Governor Ronald Reagan closed the hospital for lack of enrollment.

Word of the Mendocino Plan's "financial success" spread rapidly. Almost immediately, the federal government adopted this pilot program nationwide and tens of thousands of mental patients were de-institutionalized, contributing largely to the homeless population. The Nazis killed mental patients outright. Jones's plan of neglect had the same effect but the elements and the patients' inability to live independently in society would be their cause of death. No one suspected that the second Holocaust was beginning.

Jones needed a doctor for his experiments so he created one. As unbelievable as it is, the generally accepted story is that a young, drug addicted, vagabond wandered into the Redwood Valley compound because the *I Ching*, a Chinese book of prophesies, told him he would meet a charismatic leader there. The truth is Larry Schacht was the son of a wealthy electrical engineer from Houston, Texas who Jones recruited, if only for his namesake, or perhaps because he was actually a descendent of the notorious Dr. Hjalmar Horace Schacht, the Nazi's Minister of Economics who raised the capitol to create I.G. Farben and worked with their bankers like Hugo Philips to establish the system of concentration camps in Europe. Jones paid for Larry Schacht's pre-med education at Santa Rosa Junior College and further medical training in Guadalajara, Mexico. It was a calculated decision. Schacht returned to the US to intern in San Francisco and days before he would have received his license to practice medicine, Jones sent him to Guyana. Ultimately, Dr. Larry Schacht would mix the cyanide cocktail in Jonestown. The military Mortuary at Dover Air Force Base would later identify his body among the dead but, as we will see, their conclusions were not always correct.

It is entirely possible that Larry Schacht was related to Dr. Hjalmar Schacht. Back in the late 1920s the elder Schacht toured the United States in an effort to raise funds for the fledgling Nazi Party. He spent a great deal of time in Connecticut where he could have fathered a child. Larry's father, Ezra Schacht was born in Connecticut at about that time. One report claims that Ezra Schacht was a 'person of interest' in the FBI's investigation into the assassination of President Kennedy.

Jones's nurses operated what was recognized as the finest Sickle Cell Anemia clinic in the country. Sickle Cell Anemia is an autosomal recessive genetic disorder, similar to Tay-Sachs disease that Mengele studied.

Whereas Tay-Sachs affects descendents of Eastern European Jews, Sickle Cell Anemia affects descendents of black Africans. There will never be a cure for autosomal recessive diseases. Mengele and Jones were not looking for a cure. They were trying to better understand the genetic differences that made only these groups susceptible to the diseases so they might prey upon those differences and create a genetically specific disease that would target only these groups. Jones's nurses also experimented with electro-shock and sensory deprivation. During temple services, unruly children were brought into a side room and shocked repeatedly. Some say it was a cattle prod, others that it was a heart defibrillator and others that it was an electro-shock machine pirated from the state mental hospital. They called it "The Blue Eyed Monster." Through the public address system, the congregation heard the children's screams and cries for help. They emerged from the room groveling at Jones's feet, pleading for forgiveness.

Mendocino's population was mainly Caucasian and Jones needed blacks for his experiment. Jones's attorney, Tim Stoen, led the way when, in April of 1969, he accepted a job as director of the Legal Aide Society of Alameda County which included the predominately black population of Oakland. Stoen was positioned to offer poor black youths, in trouble with the law, a second chance at a new life in the idyllic countryside of Mendocino County under the "protection" of the Peoples Temple, and many accepted. Jones had purchased eleven used Greyhound buses in which he transported his followers to Oakland and San Francisco where he held services in borrowed churches and school auditoriums. He was careful to tone down his rhetoric and present his "church" as a multi-racial experiment in socialism that provided tangible, real world value to its followers and not some pie in the sky promise of an afterlife. He was wildly popular and amassed so many followers that he could pick and choose whomever he wanted. While in the Bay Area, the temple band played, the choir sang, and aides conducted services, all culminating in Jones's sermon, but Jones spent most of his Sundays at the Berkeley Hills home of Dr. Lawrence Layton.

Dozens of books have been published about the Layton family's contributions to Jonestown, but there is not one word about the contributions of the patriarch, Dr. Layton. Jones's personal Sunday church services were at the feet of Dr. Layton. They met, in private sessions, for several hours each Sunday, for more than two years. That is about 500 hours of meetings, obviously important to both men, but no one has ever even speculated about the subject of their discussions. Jones and Dr. Layton had only one thing in common; the creation of the perfect ethnic weapon. They were planning the Jonestown experiment.

During this period, there were ten to twelve murders committed in and around the Peoples Temple. Some victims presented obstacles to Jones's real estate acquisitions, but most were temple members who had willed their properties to Jones, only to succumb to an untimely death. Maxine Harpe was hung by an extension cord from the triangular rafters of her garage. Yes, her death scene resembled a harp and yes, after her death, Jones owned the garage and the estate it sat on. Rory Hithe was shot dead by Temple guard Chris Lewis during a heated discussion about San Francisco anti-poverty politics in an open meeting of the Western Addition Project Area Committee. Virtually, all the witnesses were temple members. Jones came to Lewis's legal defense, who was found innocent on grounds of self defense. Truth Hart was another victim. She had willed all her possessions to Jones, who proceeded to ask his nurses if there was a drug that could induce a heart attack; a heart attack that killed Truth Hart.

John Head was a patient at the Mendocino State Hospital, who suffered from depression after a motorcycle accident. He received a $10,000 insurance check that temple members encouraged him to transfer into silver bullion and donate to the Peoples Temple. Three weeks after his donation, John Head died from head injuries suffered from a fall from a three-story building. Azrie Hood just disappeared and was presumed dead. Years later, the last of what has come to be known as the "H file Homicides" occurred on October 5, 1976. Bob Houston was a member of the Peoples Temple, but resigned only to be killed the next day when he was crushed by a train car in the Oakland railroad yards where he worked.

By 1974, Jones was ready to move his operations to San Francisco and he entered triumphantly, conquering both the politics and the people.

# S I X

## THE SHALOM PROJECT

*"Why, I remember the first time I had to go into that room and tell Ryan what we were doing in Angola."*

**—Former CIA Director William Colby in a conversation with the author on April 24th, 1996, a few days before his death.**

The Shalom Project was neither Jewish nor peaceful. It was a joint effort between US and British Intelligence to train and arm Brazilian mercenaries to fight in a civil war in the South African country of Angola. Their training camp, in the remote jungles of Guyana, would eventually be the site of the Jonestown Agricultural and Medical Project.

As had been anticipated for years, in 1975 Angola won its war of independence from Portugal, only to be thrown into an internal civil war for control. It was a classic Cold War struggle; communists vs capitalists. The Soviets and the Cubans seized the opportunity and sent 10,000 troops to tip the scales in their favor, but the US was well prepared to counter the communists' offensive. Indicative of the reoccurring theme in US foreign policy, the real issue here was Angola's vast off-shore oil reserves.

Angola had been a Portuguese colony for so many years that the native black Africans spoke Portuguese. In order for the US to infiltrate the Angolan society, it needed Portuguese speaking blacks and the only other place in the world where that combination could be found was in Brazil. The Brazilian government allowed the US to recruit its military and ex-military, but prohibited it from conducting any other activities on their soil. They cherished their 'plausible deniability,' but their concerns were misplaced. They allowed CIA operatives like Jim Jones to recruit mercenaries from their military ranks, but failed to see that Jones and the CIA were also organizing their military for a planned CIA-backed coup that successfully toppled the Brazilian government just two years later. Now it was time for the new Brazilian military government to reciprocate and provide the mercenaries that Jones had identified and the CIA needed in their war in Angola.

The project was headed by naval intelligence commander, Admiral Charles Buford, but he did not have autonomous control. Ever since the CIA had helped steer the transition of power from British Guiana to Guyana, they had always worked hand in hand with their British counterparts and this project was no exception. Enter British agent George 'Phil' Blakey.

It was not by chance that Deborah Layton met Phil Blakey in England and brought him back to the United States to join the Peoples Temple. It was all by design; Blakey was the British MI6 representative in the Shalom Project.

Jones had Blakey arrange to lease several thousand acres of uninhabited jungle from the government of Guyana starting in 1973, but did not sign the five-year lease until late 1975, but the original dates were not revised. It is this two-year period between 1973 and 1975 that Jones basically controlled the land, but his name was not on the lease or associated with Shalom. So, the lease was set to expire in December, 1978, just one month after Jonestown's demise. Even as early as 1973, the final schedule may have already been set.

The location of the operation was strategically placed. Jones met with two American advisors to the Guyana National Service charged with developing the interior. They were probably CIA, but regardless, they agreed on a very remote, uninhabited tract of land in the northwest. It was thirteen miles from the Venezuelan border, which was critical because Guyana and Venezuela had a long-standing border dispute and an American outpost so close to the border would certainly deter the Venezuelans from invading. The site was fifteen miles from Port Kaituma with its airstrip and river port that lead to the ocean. In the other direction, it was twenty miles from an old rail head at Mathews Ridge. With air, sea, and rail transportation at hand, the site was perfect, but for one obstacle: there was still fifteen miles of dense jungle between Port Kaituma and the proposed site. They needed to build a road.

Phil Blakey was appointed logistics officer in charge of the nine or ten administrators that Jones initially sent to Guyana. Blakey was a licensed sea captain and Jones purchased a 65-foot ocean-going ship for him to transport the troops from Brazil to Guyana, but *The Albatross* did not solve the problem. There was still fifteen miles of jungle in the way. There were two other ships- *The Cudjo*, a fishing trolley, and *The Marceline*, that looked so much like *The Albatross* that it could have been the same ship sailing under a different name to deceive the authorities. Jones had registered all three ships in Panama. Blakey still needed to blaze a trail, but had no experience with earth moving equipment, so Jones set up a classroom where Blakey could learn to operate bulldozers, backhoes, and other large earth moving equipment. He would dig a swimming pool at the Berkeley Hills, California home of Dr. Lawrence Layton.

The actual mercenary training was done by 200 US special forces troops, some of whom stayed on to be the Jonestown guards.

The goal was to bolster a rag-tagged group of undisciplined, marijuana smoking Angolan rebels known as UNITA. UNITA was the CIA's only hope in the conflict. They needed guidance and weapons; a lot of weapons. The CIA turned to their resident arms dealer, Frank Terpil. Terpil lived about two miles from CIA headquarters in Langley, Virginia. His hands and guns were in about every CIA covert operation in Africa. He was notorious for his support of, and friendship with, Ugandan Dictator Idi Amin, a connection that would later allow Jones to escape at least as far as Uganda. Years later, Terpil's work landed him in serious legal trouble that may or may not have been related to this story. When his pleas to the CIA for help went unanswered, Terpil fled to England. In a BBC documentary entitled "The Most Dangerous Man in the World," Terpil revealed his role in Jonestown to the interviewer. It was his attempt to blackmail the CIA to come to his aid, or he would expose their involvement in the Jonestown experiment. Terpil left the television studio and has not been seen since.

Phil Blakey completed the swimming pool in Berkeley and the road in Guyana. He cleared the jungle settlement, built a saw mill, a few rudimentary cabins, and a short wave radio shack. All radio communications were coded. At a predetermined time and frequency, a conversation would begin, A code word signaled a frequency change, and the conversation would continue at that new frequency, preventing any eavesdroppers from hearing more than just partial sentences. The practice is illegal, but next to impossible to police. Much of the FBI's solid evidence on the internal workings of Jonestown was provided by members of the "Amateur Radio Relay League" who monitored Jonestown's radio communications in objection to their illegal use of the airwaves. Their contributions were priceless.

Phil Blakey stayed with the project through the final days of Jonestown, but he never had much to do with Jones, the Peoples Temple, Jonestown, or the experiments. He spent most of his time at sea or living aboard *The Albatross,* at the Port Kaituma dock. Someone had to guard the ship. The locals had a reputation for stealing anything that was not nailed down and a few things that were. In the final days, Blakey sailed to Port-au-Prince, Haiti and back to the Port of Spain, Trinidad, where he received an un-encoded radio communication from Jonestown instructing him to pick Jones up at the mouth of the Waini River. Blakey did not pull anchor and remained in Trinidad. He knew that it was a diversion. Jones was headed in the opposite direction. Authorities confiscated the ship and briefly detained Blakey, but he was released to return, not to the US or back to England, but to Angola to continue his mission.

Congressman Leo Ryan leaked word of the CIA's involvement in the Angolan Civil War to CBS news man Daniel Schorr and it caused months of embarrassment to the CIA, that eventually was denied funding for the project by Congress.

There is an interesting footnote to the location selected for Shalom and Jonestown. Originally, the Nazis did not want to kill the Jews, they just wanted to remove them from Europe. Their initial plan was to relocate the Jews to Madagascar, an island off the east coast of Africa, but this proposal proved to be too expensive. Extermination was cheaper. After World War II, the United States had a similar plan to relocate the surviving Jews to Sitka, Alaska, where they could find a safe haven and help the US develop this virgin territory. Britain's plan was to relocate the surviving Jews to the Northeast territory of British Guiana to help them develop their struggling colony. The site they selected was exactly the same one that Jones selected years later. As a student of history, the irony could not have escaped Jones.

# SEVEN

## BRACE YOURSELF, SAN FRANCISCO

*"When it came to winning elections in San Francisco, forget it without Jones."*

**—San Francisco District Attorney Joe Freitas.**

In the early 1970s, Jones and his troops advanced on San Francisco. Their siege took about two years, but in the end, they owned the city. First, he purchased another former Jewish synagogue for his headquarters on Geary Street. Jones, his aides Tim Stoen and Mike Prokes, George Moscone, Joe Freitas, and city officials had several private meetings intended to change the voter registration laws. Under the new regulations, registered voters received a receipt to produce at the polling place, but were not required to surrender that receipt, and so could vote at any and all of the city's 1,200 polling places. Jones made certain that everyone in his congregation was registered and on election day in 1975, he bussed hundreds from one polling place to the next. As instructed, they voted for George Moscone for mayor, Joe Freitas for district attorney, and Dianne Finestein and Art Agnos for city supervisors. All of them won, but Jones underestimated voter turnout, and more votes were cast than there were registered voters; an obvious indication of fraud. The public demanded an investigation and the person appointed to conduct that investigation was none other than Jones's attorney, Tim Stoen. Stoen's final report never mentioned Jones and ultimately reached no conclusions.

Also on the ballot for city supervisor was a relatively political unknown named Harvey Milk. Milk was a self-avowed homosexual who had moved from New York City to the sexual freedom of San Francisco. To the rest of the world, San Francisco was a haven for gay men. To San Franciscans, that haven was the Castro District. Milk owned and operated the Castro Street Camera Shop, and his work as a neighborhood activist soon earned him the unofficial title of "Mayor of Castro Street." During the campaign, Jim Jones phoned Milk to offer volunteers in the Western Addition and Tenderloin districts of the city. Jones asked for 30,000 copies of Milk's literature, and despite the fact that this was all Milk had, or could afford, he agreed. He knew he had strong support in the Castro, but this was a city-wide election, and he needed other neighborhoods to win. Milk's campaign managers argued against it. "Jones is supporting Agnos, and now he wants to help us?" Milk's position was that Jones was hedging his bets. "Fuck him," he said. "We'll take his volunteers and give him nothing in return." Two of Milk's campaign workers, Tory Hartmann and Tom Randol, were instructed to deliver the literature to Sharon Amos at the temple's Geary Street headquarters. When they arrived, a guard at the door insisted they put the literature in the alley. This was valuable cargo to them, so they demanded to deliver it inside. Reluctantly, the guard agreed and they brought the boxes inside. What they saw was a hallway with many doors, and outside of each door stood an armed guard. They returned to Milk to report that the building looked more like CIA headquarters than a church. As for Jones's help, there was none. He instructed his people to dump the literature into the trash. Milk lost the election, but he stayed politically active, waiting for the next election in 1977.

For his efforts, Mayor Moscone appointed Jones, Director of the San Francisco Housing Authority, an extremely lucrative position. Now he could place his indigent followers in publicly-funded housing and glean all of their government support checks, but there was a problem. Too many of his followers were being robbed as they left the bank and walked through the crime infested Tenderloin neighborhood on their way to give Jones their cash. Jones petitioned the federal government to electronically transfer his followers' support checks directly into his account. This was a novel idea at the time and the birth of what we know today as 'direct deposit.' A lifetime Republican, Jones found it necessary to reregister as a Democrat to facilitate his appointment from a Democratic mayor. In 1979, in the aftermath of Jonestown, federal and state officials investigated Tim Stoen's handling of the 1975 election fraud but failed to prove anything because all voting records were missing from a safe in city hall.

After the 1975 elections, Jones became increasingly political. With his public persona of a radical socialist, he easily attracted left-wing activists like Angela Davis, Dick Gregory, Eldridge Cleaver, Dennis Banks, Jane Fonda, Tom Hayden, and Cesar Chavez, all of whom were guests of Jones and confided in him, only to have their inner-most thoughts and plans forwarded to the CIA. The CIA had just engineered a right-wing military coup in Chile that resulted in the death of elected President Salvatore Allende. They succeeded, but there were loose ends that Jones was tasked to tie up. He invited the fallen president's widow, Laura Allende, and Chile's former finance minister for an extended visit in San Francisco. He gleaned as much inside information from them as he could and then frightened them by showing CIA torture films taken on a ship anchored off the Chilean coast. The films depicted unspeakable acts like a woman being continually raped by trained attack dogs and a pregnant woman given a Caesarean section without anesthesia while her husband was forced to watch the painful death of his wife and child. Mrs. Allende should have questioned how Jones had come to possess such classified films. Mainstream politicians like Walter Mondale and Rosalyn Carter also visited Jones in San Francisco. His ability to turn out the troops in an election was gaining a reputation.

Meanwhile, Supervisor Dianne Finestein had an uphill battle getting any legislation passed through the Board of Supervisors. She continually fell one vote short until the 1977 elections.

By 1977, Jones was in Guyana and his influence in San Francisco politics had seriously diminished. Moscone and Feinstein were reelected, but so was Milk, due largely to a change from city-wide elections to neighborhood elections. The public life of the nation's first openly homosexual elected official was not without its problems or dangers. Milk started receiving death threats in the mail. At first, he was alarmed, but, as they increased, he became more accustomed to them, except for one. Someone had broken into his apartment and spray painted, "Beware the Idles of March" on his kitchen wall. It struck him as being both extremely vague, yet extremely specific. On March 15th, Milk set out for work at city hall. He remained at work for about an hour past close of business, perhaps reluctant to leave the security he felt in city hall. Eventually, Milk made his way home to his roommate and partner Jack Lira. As Milk opened his front door, he was greeted by a mystery; a trail of voter registration cards and anti-gay brochures lead him from the living room, through the dining room, the kitchen, the bedroom, and onto a covered rear porch. There was a black curtain hanging from the ceiling. When Milk pulled back the curtain, he was horrified to discover the lifeless body of his lover, Jack Lira, hanging from a noose attached to the roof rafters. Nailed to the rafter was a transcript of the television series *Holocaust*. Milk cut Lira down, and ran to a nearby fire station for help, but they could not revive him.

Lira's death was deemed a suicide, It was front page news, but only for a day. Both the police and the press treated the death very gingerly, respecting Milk's loss. Milk received hundreds of cards and letters of condolence, but none were more interesting than the fifty, nearly identical letters he received from Jonestown. Temple aide Sharon Amos, wrote, "I had the opportunity in San Francisco when we were there to get to know you and thought very highly of your commitment to social actions and to the betterment of your community. I hope you will be able to visit us here some time in Jonestown. Believe it or not, it is a tremendously sophisticated community, though it is in a jungle." Jones was positioning himself as a friend. Eight months later, he would order Milk's assassination.

There was a battle being fought on the San Francisco Board of Supervisors. On one side of the conflict was Diane Finestein, representing the interests of wealthy real estate developers. On the other side was Harvey Milk, who advocated neighborhood control of the city. Finestein tipped the scales in her favor by running a patsy for another seat on the board. She chose a political unknown named Dan White. White was an extremely ridged, right wing, robotic, humorless fireman with a questionable history. He was a Vietnam veteran and a San Francisco policeman, living beyond his means in a Sausalito houseboat and driving an expensive sports car, but then something happened. He resigned from the police force, moved out of the houseboat, sold his car, and disappeared for one year. No one has ever accounted for Dan White's "missing year" but many have speculated he was a subject of brainwashing by a higher agency of law enforcement. Dan White was very strange. At meetings, he would seem to fall into a trance and then goose step march around the room. This was a very disturbed individual.

Finestein failed to tell her naive prodigy that, once in office, due to a conflict of interest, White needed to resign his well-paid fireman's job in exchange for a token salary as a city supervisor. He was devastated to discover he could no longer support his pregnant wife. Finestein arranged for White to be given a lucrative food concession at Pier 39, a tourist attraction being developed by her real estate backers, and that additional income forestalled the inevitable.

White was making so much money from the "Hot Potato" concession that he resigned as city supervisor but, rescinded his resignation a few days later after meetings with "law enforcement officials" just as Congressman Ryan was arriving in Guyana but Moscone and Milk would not accept him back on the board. They thought that Finestein, who Milk openly referred to as "The Wicked Witch of the West," just wanted her deciding vote back. It was a political battle. The local Nazi Party supported "Gentle Dan" as they called White.

Meanwhile, Milk's political career was blossoming. He managed to get a bill on the agenda of the board's next meeting that would have approved funding for a San Francisco gay cultural center. He was also planning a nationwide gay march on Washington scheduled for the following spring.

A few weeks before Jonestown, Harvey Milk did everything that he could to convince Congressman Leo Ryan not to visit Jonestown, but when his pleas fell on deaf ears, Milk wrote a letter to President Jimmie Carter asking for his help to stop Ryan from walking into a CIA trap. Milk was in as much trouble with the CIA as was Ryan.

About a week after the White Night destruction of Jonestown, Dan White stayed up all night pondering his problems and allegedly eating sugary pastries. The next morning, supposedly on a sugar high, he stumbled through city hall and does not remember anything about the assassinations that occurred. At the time, city hall was under construction. There were unfamiliar workmen everywhere. Among them was a CIA assassin. He first shot Moscone, once in the head, and then proceeded to Milk's office. Milk knew that he would soon be killed for knowing that Jones was CIA, so he spent his last week settling the business of his life. He closed his camera shop, turned in his leased car, and amended his will to request that several packs of Kool-Aid be spread on the Pacific Ocean with his ashes. Among other things, he met with an acquaintance, an airline pilot, named Carl Carlson, who had offered to loan Milk the money he needed to consolidate his debts. At least Milk knew this was a bad investment. He was planning his own death. Mr. Carlson was in Milk's office typing the loan agreement when he claims Dan White asked to see Milk in White's former office where Milk was shot dead, once in the head.

With all the construction noise, no one heard the gunshots. The only people who actually saw Dan White in city hall were the mysterious Carl Carlson and Dianne Finestein who claimed to have seen White pass by her open office door.

The real assassin had easy access, dressed as a construction worker with a gun in his toolbox, while White just walked through city hall in a daze. In the basement, another group of agents were busy rifling through records looking to steal any evidence of the 1975 elections that Stoen might have overlooked.

Meanwhile, White went about his business, but turned himself in to his old police station, when he learned that he was wanted by the authorities. He could not even remember being in City Hall.

Dianne Feinstein was the first to jump on the political bandwagon and publicly profess that Jim Jones and the CIA had nothing to do with the assassinations. She was answering rumors that were circulating throughout San Francisco, but she needed to do more. She appointed Dr. Chris Hatcher, and for the next twenty years, his job was to council survivors and relatives of victims of both Jonestown and the Moscone/Milk assassinations. Everything he learned was reported back to Feinstein. From Bonn, Germany, President Ronald Reagan called a press conference in which he said Jonestown was "a horrible thing, almost without precedent," and that the assassinations of Moscone and Milk were "an individual thing." "An individual thing?" Why would "The Great Communicator" feel compelled to say that? Was he trying to dispel rumors or was he trying to hide the truth?

In the opening arguments at White's trial, Attorney Dough Schmidt linked Jonestown to the assassinations, but he was quickly silenced and the subject was never breached again. The only evidence presented was testimony from Diane Feinstein and Carl Carlson that Dan White was seen in city hall when Moscone and Milk were murdered.

White was sentenced to two counts of voluntary manslaughter, after a successful defense on the grounds of "diminished capacity"; in other words, the former policeman had eaten too many doughnuts. No longer allowed in California courts, the "Twinkie defense" spurred riots in the streets of San Francisco. The "White Night Riots" were the worst the city had ever suffered. San Francisco's gay community went on a rampage, attacking city hall, setting fire to dozens of police cars, and inflicting millions of dollars in damages. White received a short sentence in a minimum security, 'country club' prison, complete with conjugal visits. Once released, White was not safe in San Francisco. He planned to move to Ireland and traveled there to make arrangements, but died when he returned to retrieve his family. On October 21,1985, White was found dead of carbon monoxide poisoning in his garage. Police investigators would say only, "Look at the running car and the hose from the tailpipe and draw your own conclusions." Conclusions should have been drawn not from his death, but from his life. Dan White was a patsy who was set up and framed for killing Moscone and Milk.

With Moscone dead, Finestein was appointed mayor of San Francisco. She controlled every aspect of the investigation into the Peoples Temple and the assassinations of Moscone and Milk. Eventually, she was elected senator from California.

In the months that followed, the CIA managed to whittle away at their reporting requirements as specified in the Hughes-Ryan Amendment. They were no longer required to provide full disclosure to six committees of Congress, only partial disclosure to three committees and full disclosure to just one elected individual. Out of 315 million US citizens there is only one person entrusted with the secrets of the CIA; the Chairperson of the US Senate's Intelligence Committee who, as of this writing, is none other than California State Senator Dianne Finestein. In a relatively short time, CIA oversight had come full circle and they were once again free to run amuck.

# E I G H T

## IT'S A JUNGLE OUT THERE

*"If God aides me to settle Guiana, Trinidad will be the richest trade center in the Indies, for if Guiana was one-twentieth of what it was supposed to be, it would be richer than Peru."*

**—Sir Walter Raleigh in 1593, after he had explored the Northeast shoulder of South America.**

With reports like this and others, European capitals set out on a massive land grab of the Northeast coast of South America. France took a tract they called French Guiana. The Dutch took Dutch Guiana (now called Surinam) and after a brief failed attempt by the Netherlands, Britain took the largest area, the size of the State of Idaho, that they called British Guiana (now known simply as Guyana). There was no need for an invading army or conflict of any kind. The region was so sparsely populated that they only had to unload their ships and claim ownership. The few indigenous Carobs just retreated back into the jungle. The British planted a flag on the beach and declared sovereignty over a long coastline and all the hinterlands, in other words, all the interior lands drained by the rivers that crossed that beach into the ocean, but not even they knew what that encompassed. Surveys were commissioned and approximate boundaries established, but they were only arbitrary lines sketched on a map of the jungle. It was all open to interpretation.

Vast fortunes were at stake. Guiana was rich in precious stones, diamonds, gold, bauxite, manganese, and timber, but with its climate, rainfall, soil and two or three growing seasons, agriculture had the greatest potential. The British imported African slaves and East Indian indentured servants to toil in their rice and sugarcane fields, all of which were near the coast. They named their seaside capital Georgetown, after the King of England, and were the only country in South America to designate English as the official language.

In Sir Walter Raleigh's time, "Guiana" encompassed parts of Venezuela as well. A major problem arose in 1821 when Venezuela achieved its independence and challenged its border with British Guiana. In 1840, a British surveyor published a map, that gave all the disputed territory to Britain. The

Venezuelans immediately protested the loss of what their maps called "Venezuela Esperia." England stalled for forty years while they tried and failed to fortify the border. In 1886, Venezuela broke off diplomatic relations with Britain and looked to the US for help to resolve the dispute. In 1895, the US Congress passed a resolution calling for arbitration, which along with a strong note from the Secretary of State, was sent to London. Britain continued to stonewall Venezuela and the US until President Grover Cleveland convinced Congress to allocate the then astronomical amount of $100,000 for a Parisian board to resolve the dispute. In 1899, the French determined that all the disputed land belonged to Britain. And so it remained until 1966, when, tempted by the weakness of the new independent government of Forbes Burnham, Venezuela resurrected its land claim, sighting evidence of collusion between Britain and the supposedly independent French arbitrators. Surinam, to the south, had a similar claim, that together put Guyana at risk of losing over 80 percent of its land.

Venezuela immediately invaded Guyana's Northeast territory and occupied the river island of Ankoko that Guyana claimed was half theirs. A few years earlier, a ten pound gold nugget was found on the island. Fortunes were in the balance.

More important than its mineral wealth was the region's potential for hydroelectric power production on the Upper Mazaruni River that would rival the largest dam in the world. With nearby natural resources and cheap power to convert them into finished goods, the region had the potential to become a major manufacturing center. Venezuela coveted the land, but was reluctant to aggressively take it because Russia had grown to be its largest trading partner and it was widely accepted that the United States had put Guyana's Prime Minister Burnham into power. The Venezuelans did not want the Cold War to be played out on their soil. An all out Venezuelan invasion was narrowly averted in 1970, when under pressure from the US, Venezuela signed the Port-of-Spain Protocol agreeing to forego their land claim for twelve years to see what, if anything, Guyana could do to develop its Northwest territory.

Guyana's problem was simple. They could not claim ownership to land they did not occupy. Ninety-five percent of the population lived on the coast that comprises only 5 percent of the country. Five percent of the population lived on the remaining 95 percent of the inland territory and most of them were apolitical, primitive natives who were too preoccupied with surviving the harsh conditions of the jungle to participate in government. The people of Guyana were not pioneers. They preferred to live on the coast and look across the sea to their Caribbean Island neighbors for their identity. They thought of themselves as Caribbeans, not South Americans. They never ventured into the remote interior of their own country. The jungle was teeming with dangers. The largest, man eating jaguars in the world lay in ambush in the trees. With one bite, they can crush a man's skull and drag him by the head back up the tree—not a settling thought as one walks through the dense jungle. There are bird-eating spiders as big as dinner plates, brightly colored frogs poisonous to the touch, 350 pound anaconda snakes, so large that they can strangle and swallow a man whole. Even the little foot long Coral snake is among the most poisonous in the world. The waters are even worse, full of blood-sucking leaches, piranhas, electric eels that packed a 500-volt punch capable of stunning and drowning a man, and the very deadly black caiman, a prehistoric relative of the crocodile. Surrounding everything is the ever present invisible threat of malaria and typhoid fever. Guyana's interior is still one of the most inhospitable regions in the world. It is so isolated that, even to this day, there are no roads or railway lines connecting it to any of its three adjacent neighboring countries.

Every government in the world recognized that Burnham was a puppet of the CIA. The true seat of power in Guyana was the quasi-government of the CIA in the US Embassy. Guyana and/or the CIA had a problem and Jim Jones was the solution. Together they created the "Guyanese National Service," a Hitler youth type program, to establish military-like encampments in the interior to further development. Enlistment in the national service was not mandatory however, without it, a young person was barred from the country's only university and all but the most menial jobs. After three years into the project, it was obvious that it was failing miserably. Apathy was as common as expertise was scarce. The fledgling new CIA backed government of Guyana needed a successful example of how to develop its interior lands and Jonestown provided it.

From the very beginning, the Jonestown pioneers sent extremely detailed weekly reports to Prime Minister Burnham about their progress. Every board, every nail, every project or process was meticulously documented. It started with the construction of the road to Jonestown that Phil Blakey carved from the jungle, three or four times as wide as it needed to be. The extra land kept the jungle at bay, but it also created two fifteen mile long narrow farm fields. They planted bananas, citrus, pineapple, and the local mainstay, cassava, on the roadside, which made it very easy to care for. The tractor was only a few feet away on the road. Harvesting was even easier. The tractor pulled a trailer loaded with fifty-five gallon drums of water. Workers dug the cassava roots and walked only a few feet to throw them into the barrels. The jostling action of the trailer along the bumpy dirt road washed the roots and by the time they reached the processing mill, they were clean. This eliminated the most labor intensive step in cassava production. It was American ingenuity at its best and something totally foreign to the Guyanese.

The Jonestown settlers constructed a saw mill to turn the local timber into structural lumber and so mastered the art that they were able to build and furnish cabins with only the import of tin roofing, nails, and paint. They took discarded fifty-five gallon drums, cut them in half, and welded them in a pinwheel design that turned on an axis in the wind. The power generated was linked to an old car alternator that charged a bank of batteries. An inverter converted the power from DC to AC to provide electricity for the short wave radio shack underneath. It was essential that the radio shack had its own dedicated power source. The rest of Jonestown relied on electricity provided by methane gas. All the excrement from the farm animals and the residences produced methane gas to power a converted generator that created electricity for the community at large. Food scraps were placed in bins filled with red worms that composted the matter into worm casings that are the "Black Gold" of gardeners.

The "Jonestown launderette" was state-of-the-art with hot water from the sun and drying by wood fired clothes dryers as air drying was unreliable due to more than 100 inches of annual rainfall, which also made for a muddy mess that was resolved with the addition of raised wooden sidewalks throughout the community. Of all their innovations, Jones was most proud of his solar powered hot water showers. Pipes were run in a serpentine pattern over the tin roof of the bath house and everything was painted black Just as the sun heats the interior of a car on a hot summer day, the sun heated the water in the pipes that rose to the holding tank above that provided free hot showers in the outback of the jungle. Jonestown was truly a self-sustainable community, that provided Burnham's government with the quintessential example of how to settle the interior. The temple pioneers had overcome every obstacle the jungle presented with only a few exceptions. They found that if they left the tractor in the field overnight, in the morning, they were greeted by a jaguar sitting in the driver's seat, sampling the human scent and waiting for his opportunity.

Jonestown's contribution to the security of Guyana's interior is best described by Laurence Mann, Guyana's Ambassador to the United States, in a letter he wrote to his foreign minister in 1977:

"We have not, of course, told the press that the peopling of the North-west region of the country near the Venezuela front by American citizens is a consideration not to be dismissed lightly, since the death of American citizens in a border war cannot be a matter of indifference to the Department of State. Nor have we told the press that Bishop Jones's endorsement of the party, the government, and its philosophical objectives is not a matter of regret to us."

A month before the massacre, in October 1978, Jonestown was at its most impressive and Jones informed Prime Minister Burnham that it was time to resolve the Venezuelan problem.

Eight years into their twelve year Port-of-Spain protocol agreement, Burnham invited Venezuelan President Carlos Andres Perez for a state visit to Georgetown. On the flight to Georgetown, Perez's plane flew so low over Jonestown that it startled the residents. Burnham's presentation to Perez consisted of only one thing: a documentary film on Jonestown with a tour conducted by Jones himself. In the community's pantry, Jones even pointed out the stored Kool-Aid to the camera. He knew exactly what was coming the following month. US State Department officials convinced Perez that it would be suicide to invade Guyana with over a thousand Americans on the border and they coerced him into immediately making a public statement dropping all claims to the disputed territory and offering Guyana help to build the Mazaruni River dam in exchange for inexpensive electricity for Venezuela. Jim Jones had accomplished what powerful countries, international commissions, and 157 years of high-level negotiations had failed to do. He single handedly secured Guyana's interior.

In the days immediately following the White Night, all of Jonestown's communications and reports to Georgetown were gathered together and burned, leaving not a single trace of the project's contributions to Guyana.

# N I N E

## AIR CUBANA FLIGHT 455

*"The friends of the CIA, the people that are harbored by the CIA, the people that have been encouraged by the CIA, the people who had guns from the CIA to invade Cuba in 1961 are responsible"*

**—Guyana Prime Minister Forbes Burnham reacting to the sabotage of Air Cubana Flight 455.**

Jim Jones visited Guyana in early October, 1976, to check on Jonestown's progress and within hours of his arrival in Georgetown, he became embroiled in and perhaps responsible for a major international incident.

Two bombs exploded in the baggage compartment of Air Cubana Flight 455 shortly after taking off from Barbados. The plane crashed in the sea and all 73 passengers were killed. The flight originated in Georgetown, Guyana and was scheduled to fly to Havana, Cuba, via stops in Trinidad, Barbados, and Jamaica. On board were 11 Guyanese; some were government officials, including the wife of Guyana's ambassador to Cuba, who Prime Minister Burnham had instructed to take that particular flight. Also on board were five North Korean "diplomats," but among them was a camera man. The group looked more like a news crew than a delegation. Also killed were twenty-four members of the Cuban Fencing Team returning home, after winning all the gold medals at the Central American/Caribbean championship, and a few Cuban government officials assigned to their sports program.

Everyone involved blamed the CIA, including, to some extent, the CIA itself, when it openly admitted to having prior knowledge of the bomb plot. In Havana, Fidel Castro held an open air memorial service for the victims. He told the crowd of over one million in the square that, "The CIA is behind all these deeds." Washington escalated the tensions further by delaying several days before reluctantly sending condolences to Burnham at his country's loss. The US Department of State sent a strong note of protest to Burnham for his accusations of US involvement. To back up their indignation, the US charge' in Guyana, John Blacken, was recalled to Washington. Even Henry Kissinger entered into the fray to counter that Castro and Burnham's accusations of CIA complicity were, "bold faced lies." Three months later, and a few days into the new Carter administration, Blacken was sent back to Guyana to resume normal diplomatic relations.

Two Venezuelans, Freddy Lugo and Herman Ricardo Lozano, were arrested and charged with sabotage. They had booked a ticket through to Havana, but exited the plane in Barbados. They claimed to be following orders from Luis Posada and Orlando Bosch. Posada was the Director of the Venezuelan Secret Police and had been on the CIA's payroll since 1965. Posada and Bosch were promptly arrested. All countries involved convened to determine jurisdiction. It was decided that Venezuela should try the four because they were Venezuelan citizens.

At first, all four were acquitted in military court, but Venezuelan officials questioned the military's jurisdiction and the four were retried in criminal court. Scapegoats Lugo and Ricardo were found guilty. Each were sentenced to twenty years. Bosch was acquitted on a technicality, but Posada was found guilty, which presented a problem for the CIA because it was widely known that he was in their employ. What ensued were two failed prison breaks and a third successful one on the eave of his sentencing. It has been reported that the guards were bribed, obviously from the outside. Posada illegally entered the US through Texas. Venezuelan arrest warrants were suppressed and he was granted US citizenship. Otto Reich, the US ambassador to Venezuela, assisted Bosch in immigrating to the US, but Bosch was arrested on a parole violation immediately upon arriving. President and former CIA Director, George H. Bush, pardoned Bosch of all charges, despite his own Defense Department's objections that Bosch was "the most deadly terrorist working in the hemisphere."

On the day after the bombing, Jim Jones entered the Georgetown offices of the **Guyana Chronicle**. Despite the rather busy news day, Jones was granted a one hour interview in which he told reporters that he was the CIA's target on Flight 455. He produced a copy of his ticket and claimed he even went so far as to check his baggage, but refused to board the plane because he had a premonition that the CIA was going to kill him. "They tried to kill me three times in the US," he told the reporters who proceeded to write a glowing article about the "almost martyr."

There **was a reason** to bomb Flight 455. Someone on board was the target, but who? It might have been the North Koreans, who may have learned something in Guyana they were not supposed to know. It could have been the wife of Guyana's Ambassador to Cuba, or maybe she was just added to an already doomed flight. It could have been an attempt to demoralize the Cubans at the loss of their award-winning fencing team. Of all the possible targets, the truth lies not in those we know, but in those we do not know. The Cuban passenger manifest meticulously identifies only forty-eight of the seventy-three passengers. The remaining twenty-five are lumped into an unidentified category that Cuba called, "crew." According to the manufacturer, this particular Douglas DC-8 aircraft requires a crew of three. These were short, puddle-jumping flights that took less than an hour. There was not enough time to serve a meal, and even if drinks and snacks were served, two stewardesses would have sufficed. That would require a total crew of five; not twenty-five. There are twenty people unaccounted for. It is difficult to believe that the prized fencing team would travel without security, perhaps elite security, or that Cuba would miss the opportunity to conduct an intelligence gathering junket under the guise of a sporting event. The truth may never be known, but the targets would appear to be the unidentified twenty, if only because Cuba suspiciously elected not to identify them.

Burnham may have blamed the CIA in order to divert attention from the fact that he had sent the wife of his Cuban ambassador to her death. As far as Jones was concerned, at best, he used the incident to distance himself from his CIA sponsors just prior to embarking on a CIA sponsored experiment in Guyana. At worst, Jones murdered seventy-three people with a bomb in his suitcase.

In what might be a related story, a few days earlier in San Francisco, Jones chaired a meeting of his planning commission. He passed a note around the table that read, "We now have the last part we need for the bomb." Some understood the note, others were perplexed, but enough of them survived to report the incident years later. Once everyone had read it, Jones burned the note and proceeded to discuss his impending trip to Guyana. Some researchers claim that this well-documented incident was a reference to an atomic bomb, but due to its close proximity in time to Jones's trip to Guyana and the bombing of Flight 455, he was probably referring to his suitcase bomb that killed seventy-three people.

On 9/11/1977, Langley Air Force Base in Virginia reported to the FBI's Norfolk office that the day before they had monitored a suspicious radio communication from Jonestown to an undisclosed location in Venezuela in which there was a cryptic discussion of an air flight and how it might end in disaster. At that time the four defendants in the bombing were on trial and that was probably the subject of the conversation, but there may be another explanation. At this point in time, Jonestown was not even a bleep on the FBI's radar. Reports were somewhat cavalier and there were mistakes made. If the date in the FBI's files was actually a year earlier, the radio communications would have been planning the bombing of Flight 455.

# T E N

## BUILDING A VIRAL WEAPON

*"There are two things about the biological agent field I would like to mention. One is the possibility of technical surprise. Molecular biology is a field that is advancing very rapidly and eminent biologists believe that within a period of 5 to 10 years it would be possible to produce a synthetic biological agent, an agent that does not naturally exist and for which no natural immunity could have been acquired. Within the next 5 to 10 years, it would probably be possible to make a new infective microorganism which would differ in certain important aspects from any known disease-causing organisms. Most important of these is that it might be refectory to the immunological and therapeutic processes upon which we depend to maintain our relative freedom from infectious diseases."*

— Dr. Robert MacMahan of the Department of Defense to the US House of Representatives Subcommittee on Appropriations in 1970. Dr. MacMahan was seeking $10 million dollars for his project that precisely predicted the HIV virus and the AIDS epidemic. His request was granted and his time table of five to ten years proved to be very accurate. Jonestown and the outbreak of AIDS was eight years away.

*In 1972, the World Health Organization reported in their bulletin (vol. 47), "A systematic evaluation of the effects of viruses on immune functions should be undertaken... an attempt should be made to ascertain whether viruses can in fact exert selective effects on immune function ... by affecting T-Cell function as opposed to B-Cell function. The possibility should also be looked into that immune response to the virus itself may be impaired if the infecting virus damages more or less selectively the cells responding to the viral antigen ... in the relation to the immune response a number of useful experimental approaches can be visualized."*

Jonestown and the outbreak of AIDS was six years away.

During the Middle Ages, the Black Plague killed upwards of 200 million people in Europe. Everyday, the dead were piled high on carts and dumped outside the city limits, only to be catapulted back over the city walls by armies of invading Mongols. Their tactic may have been terror, but their weapon was biological. There is nothing new under the sun.

The 1970s witnessed an undeclared war fought in the chambers and corridors of Washington, D.C. between the intelligence community and a few outspoken members of Congress. On one side of the battle was the CIA and military intelligence, whose scientists were determined to continue their experiments in viral weapons on human subjects. On the other side were a few brave members of Congress who objected to their use of unwitting US citizens in medical experiments.

Congress's first volley came from Senator Sam Ervin who opened hearings to investigate CIA medical experiments on humans. Such experiments had been outlawed at the Nuremberg trials, but now the CIA with their Nazi scientists were sponsoring the same kinds of experiments in the United States that the world had so widely condemned in Nazi Germany. The CIA gave Congress a token response when it initiated a treaty with the Soviets in 1972 that banned the production, testing, and even possession of viral weapons. The treaty had no teeth. There was no verification, and both sides cheated. Next to pick up the torch was Senator Frank Church, who opened another set of hearings into the CIA's medical experiments. Senator Church bashed the CIA's **MK ULTRA** experiments with accusations that they were "rogue elephants" and "out of control." He ordered that all **MK ULTRA** files be destroyed, but it did not matter. Jones had been copying them for a decade. Senator Church's actions were well intentioned, but only served to drive the CIA's projects further underground. When Congressman Ryan set out to investigate what he thought was a CIA medical experiment in Jonestown, this was not a new issue. It was the final battle in an eight year war that Congress lost, because it focused on the civil rights violations of the test subjects and not on how the results of the experiments might ultimately be used.

It may be difficult for most Americans to accept that their government conducts lethal medical experiments on its own citizens, but just a brief study in history proves that they do, and have done so for at least the last century. Military personnel, prisoners, and the general public have long been used as "guinea pigs" to further medical science, protect national security, or advance whatever secret agenda was held by the bureaucrats who headed the projects.

A well documented example of this abuse of power was the Tuskegee syphilis experiment conducted by the US Public Health Service from 1932 until 1972, in which 600 impoverished black sharecroppers in Macon County, Alabama, were left untreated for syphilis, while doctors studied the progression of the disease as the subjects slowly died. The participants were never told that they had syphilis or the threat that imposed to their families, only that they would receive free government health care for what the doctors told them was "bad blood." They were provided transportation to examinations and a hot meal on exam days. They were also given burial insurance if they agreed to a post mortem autopsy. The subjects were never treated, not even after the 1940's when penicillin was proven to be the cure. This atrocity went unnoticed until 1972, when objections from Senators Ervin and Church prompted a front page article in the **New York Times**. Two years later, President Bill Clinton apologized, "To our Afro-American citizens, I am sorry that your federal government orchestrated a study so clearly racist." Only eight of the 600 test patients survived. Five of them attended the White House ceremony. To clean up their mess, the federal government had to compensate fifty widows and twenty children who had contracted syphilis from their husbands and fathers.

In that same year, Congress passed the National Research Act intended to prohibit medical experiments on humans, but within the rules was an exception for US federal agencies whose services were kept secret by Executive Order, in other words, the CIA.

Starting in the early 1950s, under the direction of Dr. Lawrence Layton, the US Army's Chemical and Biological Warfare Division began research into promising viral weapons that may have resulted in the AIDS epidemic. The HIV virus has been classified as a lentivirus— a small family of "slow viruses" that take a long time to incubate and are found exclusively in domesticated animals. HIV most closely resembles a combination of bovine (cattle) T-Cell Leukemia (HTLV-1) and visna (sheep) SV-4, which together mutates into the BVV virus. In 1977, scientists announced that they had successfully infected human cells with BVV and concluded that, "BVV may play a role in either malignant or slow viruses in man." **Jonestown and the outbreak of AIDS was only one year away.**

Creating the HIV virus may have been relatively simple. First, start with a purebred cow. All these experiments start with a cow because cows are extremely genetically close to humans. Infect the cow with the T-Cell leukemia virus (HTLV-1). Then, extract blood from a sheep with the SV-4 virus and inject it into the cow. Given time, the viruses will combine and mutate into BVV. Inject the cow's blood into a human and the recombinant virus will mutate further into HIV. In other words, the test person was not given HIV, only the elements for his own body to create it. This could be the one obstacle to retracing the history of HIV, because it might not have a history outside the human body. Certainly the process is more sophisticated than presented here, but with trial and error it could be replicated. The problem is that success in reproducing HIV would be followed by an arrest warrant for murder and no researcher is willing to risk that outcome.

A diagram of the spread of AIDS in the Western Hemisphere looks like a pyramid, the origins of which can be traced back to just a few gay Haitian prostitutes. Science has even pinpointed "AIDS patient 0", the one man at the top of the triangle who transmitted the virus exponentially throughout the United States. The epidemic in Africa is very different. It is heterosexual, not homosexual in origin and transmission. It started in Uganda, not with a traceable progression, but with an explosion. It was as if one day no one in Uganda was HIV positive and the next day everyone was. There may be a logical explanation. On May 11, 1987, the science editor for the **London Times**, Pearce Wright, published a front page article that claimed the World Health Organization's smallpox vaccination program in Uganda was the source of the AIDS outbreak in Africa. Doctor Robert Redfield at the Walter Reed Medical Center in Washington, D.C. confirmed Wright's allegations. Smallpox vaccinations are not given to Americans, except for new recruits into military service as a protection against biological warfare. A patient of Dr. Redfield, developed AIDS after having received a smallpox vaccination, and he was convinced it came from the vaccine. Neither of these stories, or others like it, were ever reported in the US.

Fetal calf serum is universally used to create cell tissue cultures for subsequent use in the production of smallpox vaccine. If the fetal calf serum was infected with BVV, it possessed all the elements to create HIV in anyone who received the vaccine. The vaccine had been administered in Uganda by nurses, some of whom worked for the World Health Organization, and some of whom worked for Jim Jones, who had stationed them there after Jonestown's demise.

The fact that in the entire history of mankind, AIDS first surfaced precisely at that point in time when scientists where experimenting with something that looked like AIDS, begs the question, "Did AIDS create the research or did the research create AIDS?" Since the research predates the epidemic by a few years, the later is more probable. If AIDS is finally understood and perhaps even cured, the breakthrough will come not from medical doctors or scientists, but from veterinarians. Trying to de-engineer AIDS in humans is futile, because it does not exist outside of humans. Attention should be given to the other lentiviruses in an effort to recreate HIV from the bottom up, not from the top down.

Essential to understanding HIV is the visna virus that when combined with other lentiviruses, creates the key that allows the recombinant virus to unlock the human cell and replicate. The visna virus is relatively new, having been created in a Nazi Germany viral weapons lab in the 1930s. Fearing the virus might destroy Europe's sheep population, all the infected sheep were exported to Iceland, where they could be studied in relative isolation. It did not take long before every sheep on the island was infected. The visna virus was identified and eradicated in the late 1940s and was a dead issue until the early 1970s when there was a pronounced resurgence of interest in its potential. From 1970 until 1977, public medical databases list hundreds of published experiments into the visna virus's ability to jump species, infect human beings, and act as an effective viral weapon. This extensive work all lead up to Jonestown and the outbreak of HIV in 1978.

There were only four entities in the world with the desire and resources to create AIDS— the Nazis, the old Soviet Union, the US Army's Fort Detrick facility, and Dr. Josep Mengele. The Soviets, along with their own collection of Nazi scientists, had the largest program with over 1,500 laboratories, employing thousands of researchers all looking for new ways to kill people en masse. The CIA sent agents into the Soviet Union to infiltrate these labs and at least one was caught, arrested, and deported. Jon Lodeesen was a CIA asset who taught espionage classes in a West German school for spies before being assigned to the US Embassy in Moscow, where he endeavored to glean as much information as he could about the Soviet's work in viral weaponry. Immediately after his arrest and deportation, Lodeesen traveled to Brazil, where he wrote a letter of introduction on State Department stationary to Jim Jones. The only thing these two had in common was their employer, the CIA, who obviously thought that Lodeesen had something important to offer Jones. It may have been the virus. Then there was Fort Detrick; the highest classified chemical, biological, and viral warfare lab in the world, that many believe was the origin of AIDS due to its duel interest in viral weapons and AIDS research. The lab's former director was Dr. Lawrence Layton who Jones met with weekly and whose family played such a large part in the Jonestown experiment. Dr. Layton's later work at the Western Regional laboratory of the US Department of Agriculture resembled the creation of AIDS. Back in 1974, a paper published in *Cancer Research* described how to make viruses jump species to create brand new ones. Dr. Layton fed the milk of cows infected with C-type bovine virus to newborn chimpanzees. They died a few months later from a total immune system breakdown, not from one, but from two diseases— leukemia and an opportunistic lung infection called *Pneumocystis carinii* pneumonia, neither of which had ever been seen in chimpanzees before. *Pnneumocystis carinii* combined with a cancer called Kaposi's sarcoma is today's definition of AIDS.

Finally, there was Josep Mengele, perhaps the world's foremost eugenicist and expert in blood diseases. It was Mengele who first predicted that Northern Europeans had a certain immunity to HIV because they were descendants of people who lacked a gene that allowed their ancestors to survive the Black Plague. The gene in question is the CCR5 DELTA-32. Mengele was correct. Of the millions of people infected with HIV, only **one** patient has ever been cured. The patient had been HIV positive for years and suffered from an unrelated leukemia. German scientists gave him a bone marrow transplant from a donor who was CCR5 DELTA-32 negative and it killed every HIV cell in the patient's body. The gene is the doorway into the cell and without it there is no way for the virus to enter and replicate. People who lack CCR5 Delta-32 are totally immune to HIV and AIDS. There is not one person of African, Mediterranean, or Asian ancestry who has this immunity. In the melting pot of the US, only one percent have the immunity. In the blue-eyed, blonde population of Germany, the Nordic countries and Southern Russia, upwards of five percent are protected from AIDS. Whether intentional or not, **AIDS is an ethnic weapon.** If everyone in the world were to be exposed to HIV, the only people to survive would be the Nazi's cherished Arian Race. Whether the virus was created by the Nazis, the Soviets, the US Army at Fort Detrick, or Josep Mengele, it does not matter. All roads lead back to Jim Jones.

Today, blacks are fifteen times more likely to contract AIDS than their white counterparts. Some of this discrepancy can be attributed to Blacks generally having more sexual partners than whites. They also have a higher rate of intravenous drug use. Moreover, black males are less likely to have been circumcised, which puts them at a greater risk of contracting any sexually transmitted diseases, including HIV. This is not news. Back in ancient Egypt, Bedouin tribesman suffered severe infections of the foreskin. Pharaoh's priests decreed that it was "God's will" that they be circumcised. Of course, it was not God's will, but the Bedouins accepted this more readily than if they were told it was the health code that it really was.

There are those who believe that the HIV virus evolved naturally from a monkey or chimpanzee virus, but this theory cannot be defended for two very critical reasons. First, there are no monkeys or apes in the wild that have AIDS. More important is the timing. Mankind has existed alongside other primates for millions of AIDS-free years. Against all probable odds, the outbreak of AIDS occurred precisely at that point in time when scientific knowledge of the human immune system, animal viruses jumping species, and gene splicing had advanced to a level that our elite scientists could at least grasp the concept. Had AIDS first appeared, even a few months earlier, it would have totally baffled the experts. AIDS surfaced precisely on the cutting edge of scientific research into something that looked like AIDS. Timing is everything and there is no such thing as coincidence.

AIDS is so well-engineered that thirty-five years after its onset, it is still a total mystery. Scientists cannot agree on what it is, where it originated, how to test for it, or how to cure it. There are as many theories about AIDS as there are AIDS researchers. The finest minds in the world could review everything ever written on the subject and still walk away totally confused. At the many international AIDS conferences held since 1979, scientists are repeatedly advised to "Start over" because their efforts to date have all fallen short.

Initially, researchers called the first victims of "Gay Related Immune Deficiency" the "Four H Club": Haitians, Homosexuals, Heroin users, and Hemophiliacs. AIDS is a blood disease that requires an exchange of blood in order to transmit from one person to another. With the possible exception of open sores from venereal disease, there is not usually a transmission of blood during heterosexual intercourse. It first surfaced in Haitian homosexual prostitutes who transmitted the virus to gay New York City tourists through unlubricated anal sex that often involves an exchange of some blood. The newly infected, some of whom were also heroin users, returned to the US to infect others, either through homosexual sex or shared hypodermic needles. Hemophiliacs contracted the virus from blood donated by infected members of the other groups. Once the seeds were planted, the epidemic quickly spread, but only in those groups. In these early stages, US Surgeon General C. Everett Koop warned the American public that they were at serious risk because the epidemic was about to spill over into the general population, but that never happened. AIDS is so intelligent, so precisely pinpoint accurate, that it only infects the targeted groups.

There is no test for AIDS or even HIV. There is only a test for the presence of anti-bodies created to combat HIV. To complicate matters further, it has never been proven that HIV causes AIDS. HIV **does** generally piggyback on AIDS, but it is not all inclusive. There are many people who are HIV positive who never develop AIDS, and there are those who have all the symptoms of AIDS but without HIV. Symptoms vary widely because AIDS is not a specific disease, it is a syndrome that appears to be two different diseases working in tandem; Karposi's sarcoma cancer and Pneumocystis carinrii pneumonia. Unlike other medical conditions, the diagnosis for AIDS includes the patient's lifestyle. An elderly heterosexual patient with Karposi's sarcoma will be diagnosed with cancer, while a young homosexual patient with that same affliction will be diagnosed with AIDS. So, what is AIDS? After thirty-five years, all that can be said with certainty is that AIDS is a blood disease that has killed over thirty-five million people and is growing in strength. One researcher, David Weinberg, has proposed that AIDS is not a result of the HIV virus, but was artificially created from a single human cell that he calls, "The Mengele Cell" after its inventor, Josep Mengele.

The birth and complexity of AIDS is not important. It is essential to separate the affliction from the epidemic. It is like the Chinese being credited with inventing gun powder; but did they invent anything? The elements for gun powder had existed in nature since prehistory. The Chinese just combined those elements into something useful for mankind. At some point, the secret to AIDS existed only in a test tube full of tainted human blood. Who tested it? Who used it as a weapon? Who seeded it into society? Who killed 35 million people and infected an additional 35 million to date? It does not matter who made the gun, it only matters who pulled the trigger and the trigger man was Jim Jones.

In the summer of 1978, Peoples Temple aide Terri Buford convinced attorney, Mark Lane, that Jones had some valuable information about the assassination of Martin Luther King that would help him prepare for his testimony to the House Select Committee on Assassinations hearing scheduled for later that year. Lane could not refuse, especially when Buford agreed to pay all expenses for him and his colleague, Don Freed, to travel to Guyana. While in Jonestown, as a courtesy, Jones offered them a free medical examination in the Jonestown Medical Clinic. Lane emerged with glowing accounts about the best medical exam he had ever received. Don Freed was less enthusiastic because Dr. Schacht diagnosed him with having "a fatal immune deficiency that could only have been contracted from a homosexual act." This was mid-summer, 1978, six months before the outbreak of GRID or AIDS. The first medical diagnosis of AIDS, whether right or wrong, was made in Jonestown.

# E L E V E N

## THE EXPERIMENTS

*US Senate, Ninety-fifth Congress, Hearings before the Subcommittee on Health and Scientific Research of the Committee on Human Resources, Biological Testing Involving Human Subjects by the Department of Defense, called the Pentagon to task for experimenting on US citizens. It was confirmed that 239 populated areas in the US had been contaminated with biological agents between 1949 and 1969. Pentagon spokesperson Lt. Colonel George A. Carruth was not apologetic and testified that "additional tests" would be conducted in the future if the army felt it was necessary to access our "vulnerability" to biological attacks. The year was 1977, and it should have been Congress's wake up call. The Jonestown experiments had already begun and would culminate about a year later.*

Just about every experiment conducted in the CIA's **MK Ultra** program was replicated in Jonestown. One example was sensory deprivation. In the clinical lab, the sensory deprivation chamber was a sealed box in which subjects were confined for two or three days. The human brain is a receptor designed to receive visual, audio, taste, olfactory, and tactical input. Deny the brain input and it turns in on itself and some very unusual psychological changes take place. Voodoo priests in Haiti have used this technique for hundreds of years. A subject is poisoned with a concoction containing the essence of blow fish that renders them in a coma, appearing to be dead, but still conscious of their surroundings. They are then buried alive and two or three days later, the priest would dig them up and they emerge a zombie— alive, but totally void of a brain to do any more than control heartbeat, breathing and basic motor functions. Jones borrowed this technique in Jonestown where his sensory deprivation chamber was a coffin with an air supply. Mindless zombies cannot work, which was a requirement of the experiment. The subject had to be totally void of his own will, but still capable of hard physical labor. The intent was to pinpoint the exact time in the box necessary to produce the desired results.

There were two primary experiments conducted in Jonestown; one psychological and one physical. In the first, Jones divided the representative cross section of blacks and homosexuals into different groups that received small dosages of various psychotropic drugs in order to ascertain which formula would render the subject most open to suggestion, but still capable of functioning in society. The dosages were deliberately very small so as not to be detected in routine medical examinations. The object was not to drug the subject into oblivion, but to find that delicate balance where he ceased to think for himself, could still be productive, and appeared to be outwardly healthy.

The only sugar allowed in Jonestown was in the one cookie that subjects received once a week, directly from the hand of Jim Jones. Every Sunday, all the residents lined up in the pavilion for a brief audience with "Father." As each approached his Adirondack chair throne, Jones selected a cookie from one of several containers at his side. They were required to eat the entire cookie in Jones's presence, while relating the events of their week. **One and only one cookie was the strictest rule in Jonestown.** On one occasion, a young black girl who was baking cookies in Jonestown's "Experimental and Herbal Kitchen" unaware that the cassava flour contained psychotropic drugs, handed one out an open window to her boyfriend. Temple guards, who monitored every step in the cookie production, reported the infraction to Jones. During the next Sunday gathering in the pavilion, Jones ordered the young girl and her boyfriend to disrobe and have sexual intercourse in front of the entire community. Such was the humiliating punishment for violating the "one cookie rule" and rightfully so because such deviations would contaminate the results of what was otherwise a precise experiment.

There was enough Thorazine and other mind altering drugs found in the rubble of Jonestown to supply an average US mid-sized city for over a year. The CIA's **MK ULTRA** experiments had produced some useful data, but the ultimate experiment was conducted by Jones's medical staff, who for years had used psychotropic drugs to subdue unruly mental patients at the Mendocino State Mental Hospital. Their expertise was useful, but limited to drugging mental patients into submission. The goal now was to drug mentally healthy people into submission. This extremely fine line was the reason for the first experiment in Jonestown. Residents were divided into groups, each of which received a special combination of drugs. They were required to work in the farm fields and their work was evaluated. In the end, they were subjected to the only definitive test to see whether they were under control. Jones told them to kill themselves and 403 people did.

The last thing Jones wanted was for everyone to commit suicide. The object of this exercise was to compare which formula of small dosages of which drugs would render a person more susceptible to suggestion. If everyone killed themselves, there could be no comparison. It was expected, anticipated, and even required that some residents refuse the poison and run. As with any well-designed medical experiment, there had to be a control group who received a placebo; in this case a cookie without drugs. If anyone from this group committed suicide, it would be attributed to Jones's powers of persuasion. Guards, who encircled the pavilion, tackled the runners and shot them in the back with hypodermics filled with cyanide before dragging their bodies back to the pavilion where they were placed face down in neat rows.

For months, even years, every resident had received weekly medical examinations that were well documented in extensive records of health, work performance, drugs administered, and the final entry, **Suicide Yes or No.** These records were never found in the rubble of Jonestown.

The primary experiment in mind control was designed to create sheep willing to go to slaughter, but there was a small side experiment designed to entice them to riot. Jones had devised a means to excite his audience into a wild frenzy using nothing more than the sound of the human voice. He was attempting to build on something called "Misothonia": Greek for "hatred of sound", sometimes called "Selective Sound Sensitivity Syndrome." It is a neuro-otological disorder that drives certain sensitive, otherwise normal, people into fits of murderous rage, panic, terror, fear and anger. Certain consonant, repetitive sounds can trigger this fight or flight response. It can be the sound of someone clipping their finger nails or footsteps, but it most commonly comes from the human mouth. Coughing, chewing with the mouth open or popping chewing gum can be uncontrollably detrimental to certain sensitive people. Jones attempted to perfect the exact sound that would affect everyone, not just those suffering from Misothonia. Residents were taught to flatten their dominant hand and spread their thumb and forefinger as far apart as possible. They then placed the crotch of their hand horizontally in front of their mouth and moved it back and forth rapidly as they uttered a guttural sound. It was a collectively shared mantra that literally drove them wild. Jones would make the sound first and the others would follow. The residents would violently lunge forward and then back and forward and back again as if they were attacking something that was not there. Between the sound and their reaction to it, the scene was bizarre, but perhaps not without precedent. The night before a battle, American Indian braves worked themselves into a trace-like frenzy in a war dance around the campfire by rapidly hitting their mouth with an opened hand to create a similar sound. Some Arab tribeswomen make a comparable repetitive sound with their tongue during times of celebration. Years later, in a radio interview, Deborah Layton played a tape recording of the "noise". She told the interviewer that Jones called it "Collective Effervescence", implying that he made up the name. Actually, "Collective Effervescence" (or CE) was first coined by an eminent 19th century French philosopher and founder of modern day sociology, David Emile Durkheim, who postulated that there was a wave of perceived energy that flowed over a crowd of people who shared a common experience and that energy or "groupthink" was stronger than the individual's personally held beliefs and morals. Under its influence, people would do things they would never do on their own. Examples are feelings of elevated wellness from a large religious gathering, or extreme urgency and panic felt by stampeding fans at a soccer game, or the anger and violence felt by rioters who perceived a common injustice to the group. He surmised that these shared feelings did not come from the ceremony, the soccer game or the riot, but from the people who had experienced it together. In modern terms, a man sitting home alone, watching that same soccer game on television would not share in the CE that panicked the crowd at the stadium but, if he invited a large gathering to watch the game in his home, they would develop their own CE with results entirely different from the fans in the stadium. Jones studied Durkheim's work in an effort to artificially create in his followers a groupthink of total despondency, making suicide seem attractive. In his landmark 1897 book, *Suicide,* Durkheim surmised that people do not commit suicide because something bad in the their lives had depressed them. He believed people killed themselves because of the failure of, or alienation from, their group. Durkheim theorized that a charismatic leader could induce voluntary suicide in a group if the group experienced an "abrupt change" that brought into question the individual's commitment to the group or the overall acceptance of the group into the larger society. Eighty years after the publication of *Suicide,* Jim Jones put Durkheim's theories to the ultimate, real world test. The here-to-fore accepted theory that the Jonestown mass suicides were the flippant reaction of a drug crazed cult leader are simply not true. Jones had studied the science for years. Suicide was always meant to be the end of Jonestown. He only needed a trigger or "abrupt change" in the group and the murder of Congressman Ryan provided it.

The second experiment was a purely physical study in the communicable aspects of the HIV virus. The virus was transported to Jonestown in a vile of contaminated blood. At this point, all they knew was that the human body had no resistance to the virus thanks to a few unfortunate subjects in the sub-basement of a research lab where they were surrounded by doctors in hazmat suites. They knew it was deadly, but they did not know how contagious it was. If it was an airborne pathogen or communicated by touch, releasing it could kill all of mankind. Could it be confined to just the targeted groups? Was it transmitted by saliva? A kiss? Heterosexual or homosexual sex? From mother to unborn child? They did not know as evidenced by the fact that, among the other medical supplies shipped to Jonestown, was 10,000 pairs of surgical gloves. That was the essence of the Jonestown experiment. If everything went awry, at least the contamination would be confined to the remote jungle.

Peter Waterspoon was a gay resident of Jonestown who offered oral sex to another male resident without Jones's permission. He was severely punished, heavily drugged, and placed in isolation. Such behavior may have been acceptable on the streets of San Francisco, but not in this clinical experiment.

The over 1,200 healthy test persons, or "TPs" as the Nazis called them, were assembled in an isolated environment and closely monitored. Initially, only a few were injected with the HIV virus. It was easy to follow the path of the virus through the community by following the weekly blood samples from the infected TP's co-workers, bunk mates, and sexual partners. Since sex in Jonestown, even between married couples, was prohibited except with Jones's consent and then only with observation from his medical staff, it was easy to follow the trail. It took a year to determine that they could confine it to just the targeted groups. Once he was convinced that he could control his new lethal weapon, Jones set out to deploy it.

Was Jones acting alone in his persecution of homosexuals or was this sanctioned by his CIA sponsors? It may have begun with a prejudice against gays brought into the agency by the Nazis after World War II or it might have its origins a few years later in the early 1950's during the McCarthy Era and something that has come to be known as the "Lavender Scare." Joe McCarthy was concerned that there were too many homosexuals in the intelligence community who he thought were easy targets to blackmail and force into divulging state secrets to the communists. The truth is that heterosexuals were easier targets when threatened with the lives of their spouses and children, but the State Department sided with McCarthy and set out to dismiss every homosexual they could find in the federal government. So many homosexual men were ousted from the CIA that, by the early 1960's they regrouped to form an entire community in Sausalito, California.

# T W E L V E

## THE WHITE NIGHT

*"If you gaze long into the abyss, the abyss gazes into you."*

**—Friedrich Neitzsche.**

By 1975, Angola had won its war of independence from Portugal and, as anticipated, erupted into a civil war between the communists and the capitalists for control of the new country. The last of the Shalom Project mercenaries were sent into the African conflict, vacating their Guyana encampment and making room for the first Peoples Temple pioneers. It was only at this point that Jones signed the land lease with the Guyana government that had been agreed to back in 1973.

In the first year, the Jonestown Medical and Agricultural Project was a paradise. Memories of their difficult lives in the poor neighborhoods of San Francisco and Oakland soon faded as residents enthusiastically set out to carve a new life from the jungle. They were building a town and enjoying every minute of it, that is, until Jones arrived a year later with a litany of harsh new rules and regulations to begin the experiments. Overnight, their idyllic life turned into a hell on earth; a hell that would end with something that Jones called, "The White Night."

Jones ran Jonestown as if it was an insane asylum, and to a large extent, it was. Jones was the head psychiatrist and under him was a medical doctor with a staff of nurses and guards who acted as orderlies. The residents or patients received the same anti-psychotic drugs as mental patients. The difference was they came to Jonestown sane and were driven insane by Jones. Back in his early years in Indiana, Jones had worked as an orderly in a mental hospital, where he met his future wife who worked there as a nurse. Years later, his army of nurses all worked at the Mendocino State Mental Hospital in California. Running an insane asylum was their stock in trade. It was their expertise and it was Jonestown.

Jones had spent his entire life recruiting people to join his temple, but all that stopped in Guyana. There were no Guyanese in the Peoples Temple and for good reason. Jones already had his ideal cross-section of test persons and, besides, Prime Minister Burnham had forbidden him from involving any of his citizens.

The dates on the five year lease were never changed so, even though Jones did not sign it until 1975, it was still set to expire in December of 1978. Jones originally scheduled the "White Night" for November 9, 1978 to commemorate the fortieth anniversary of the "Crystal Night," the first officially sanctioned persecution of the Jews by the German government. The date was acceptable to his CIA sponsors because they wanted to wait until after the November 3rd elections to see if Congressman Ryan was reelected or their problem just went away. Ryan was reelected, but too busy thanking his supporters back in California to meet Jones's November 9th schedule. He needed another week. Jones was more than disappointed because this postponement presented yet another problem. His original plan was to discredit his attorney Mark Lane by association prior to Lane's testimony to the House Select Committee on Assassinations Hearings that were scheduled to begin the day before Ryan would now arrive in Jonestown. The testimony of Lane and his star witness, Grace Walden, regarding the killing of Martin Luther King, would be so damaging to the CIA that it could not be allowed to proceed. The Company "finessed" the scheduling conflict by monopolizing the first day of the House hearings with testimony after testimony from CIA paid physiatrists all of whom swore that Grace Walden was not a competent witness, even before she had taken the stand. What they were really doing was stalling, waiting for a call from Jones that Ryan had arrived in Guyana. Jones would not allow Ryan in until his attorney, Mark Lane, was present. A message was sent to Lane, reminding him of his obligations and his $9,000 a month retainer, and immediately ordering him to Guyana. He stormed out of the hearings in total disgust. "You people make me sick," he said as he left Washington, D.C. for Jonestown. Grace Walden never testified. The investigation into King's assassination fell apart and the House committee moved onto their primary concern— the assassination of President John Kennedy.

During the previous year, Jones had conducted several rehearsals of the White Night in which residents were asked to drink what they were told was poison, only to find out that it was just a test of loyalty. This might have been part of the experiment and a means to adjust the drug dosages along the way or condition the test persons to accept the concept in order to produce better results. In any event, Jones never had the ability to follow through until just two days before the final White Night. Pure potassium cyanide is so lethal and guarded, that the average person cannot purchase it, but somehow

Jones managed to buy a large quantity of potassium cyanide from M & B Laboratory Chemicals in Upstate New York. It was shipped to Georgetown and transported to Port Kaituma on the *Albatross (or Marceline)*. It arrived in Jonestown just two days before the massacre. Timing is everything. There is a plausible alternate theory that Jones had established a bogus jewelry company which gave him license to purchase small quantities of cyanide used in jewelry production and that he stockpiled those shipments for over a year until he had enough. Supposedly he bought it from M & B Laboratory Chemicals in Delaware and like the first scenario, the last shipment arrived two days before the event. Apparently, the M & B company no longer exists. All attempts to locate any records of the transaction have failed.

In the few weeks before the White Night, there was an exodus of high level people from Jonestown who were a part of the experiment, but who did not want or need to be there for the end. Jones's in-laws, the Baldwins, left without explanation. Lisa Layton disappeared eighteen days earlier. Jones said she had died, but never produced a body or a grave. Top aides like Terri Buford, Paula Adams, Deborah Layton, Bonnie Malmin, and Tim and Grace Stoen all left as if they knew what was about to happen.

Back in California, ex-temple members Al and Jeannie Mills had established the Concerned Relatives Group, who were just that, concerned about their relatives in Jonestown. Deborah Layton, Bonnie Malmin, and Tim Carter, as well as Tim and Grace Stoen, who were all still working for Jones, joined the group as a vehicle to entice Congressman Ryan to investigate Jonestown. The Stoens had left their young son, John-John, in Jonestown. Jones claimed that he had fathered the boy who really did look like him. Tim Stoen had even signed an affidavit that Jones was the boy's father, but now he wanted him back. The Stoens asked Congressman Ryan to intervene in what basically was a child custody dispute.

Deborah Layton told Ryan that half of Jonestown residents suffered from severe diarrhea, extreme weight loss, skin lesions, and high fevers. Night sweats and neck stiffness were common complaints. Though it was not known at the time, these are all early symptoms of AIDS. The one witness to step forward who had the most influence on Ryan was his old friend, Associated Press photographer Sam Houston. Houston's son, Bob, was a member of the Peoples Temple until he decided to leave the fold. The next day, he was killed in the Oakland railroad yard where he worked. Sam suspected foul play, but was now concerned with his granddaughters, Judy and Patricia, who were in Jonestown. Ryan was told of other suspicious deaths of temple members. He learned of the untimely deaths of Maxine Harpe, Rory Hithe, Truth Hart, John Head, Azrie Hood, and finally his old friend Bob Houston. Back when Ryan was a school teacher in San Bruno, California, he chaperoned the school band on a trip to Washington, D.C. to play at the inauguration of President Kennedy. Bob Houston was a student in the band.

Ryan had been busy looking into the CIA's **MK Ultra** project and the possibility that Jim Jones orchestrated the kidnapping of Patty Hearst and used CIA techniques to brainwash her. While organizing his files, Ryan had an "Oh, My God!" moment when he realized that, against all probable odds, 100% of the victim's surnames began with the letter "H." There was something very seriously strange happening here and he was determined to get to the bottom of it. "The CIA Congressman," as Jones jokingly referred to Ryan, was hooked and on his way to his death in Guyana.

Jim Jones and his CIA sponsors did not do much in Guyana without the cooperation of their British counterparts in what had been their colony. The British government had little interest in Jonestown, but they **did** have an interest in the Shalom Project that preceded it. Englishman Phil Blakey had begun the project, so it was only appropriate that another Englishman clean up in the aftermath. British subject Gordon Lindsay was a reporter who investigated conflicts in Africa, especially Angola, which led him back to Jonestown. Lindsay stayed in Guyana for four months during which time he said that he investigated Jonestown, but never visited there or met Jones. When his Guyanese visa was about to expire, the US Embassy in Georgetown interceded on Lindsay's behalf to secure an extension. It is very odd that the US government would help a British subject in South America, but such was the importance of Lindsay to the CIA. According to Jones and Lindsay, the closest Lindsay ever came to Jonestown was in a privately chartered flight over the community. Jones claimed Lindsay's plane flew so low over Jonestown that it startled the residents and one elderly woman died from a heart attack. It was only Jones's propaganda, and not the facts, that established Gordon Lindsay as an enemy of the Peoples Temple.

Gordon Lindsay contacted the son of Ryan's attorney, who he knew Ryan had hired to help in his investigation. Lindsay not only recommended that Ryan travel with a contingent of reporters to Jonestown for protection, but specified which reporters to bring. Some of his recommendations had a history of investigating CIA conspiracies. Their inclusion in Ryan's party appears to be an attempt to bundle all the CIA's problems into what they knew would be their fatal trip.

Lindsay made the calls and contacts to assemble Ryan's news crew. He convinced NBC-TV to send a team headed by Don Harris with reporter, Bob Flick, cameraman Bob Brown, and soundman Steve Sung. This was NBC's veteran combat crew, having covered the Vietnam War. Harris was so close to the action that he viewed the fall of Saigon from the roof of the American Embassy. The **Washington Post** assigned their Argentina correspondent, Charles Krause. The **San Francisco Chronicle** representative was reporter Ron Javers. The **San Francisco Examiner** sent reporter Tim Reiterman and cameraman Greg Robinson. When the roster was complete, Lindsay radioed the list to Jones who forwarded it to the US Embassy in Georgetown who forwarded it to the State Department. Lindsay managed to be hired by NBC as a guide or "fixer" as they are called in the business. Excluding Lindsay, the news crew numbered eight. Only five would return alive.

The newsmen afforded Ryan some degree of protection, but he was still concerned that if they were all killed, the truth would be lost forever. He needed additional insurance policies. Ryan contacted the State Department to request information about Jonestown. For months, the State Department had been receiving hundreds of reports about Jonestown from relatives of the residents and citizens complaining about their illegal use of the airwaves and violations of US postal regulations, but they withheld this information from Ryan. Their report was no more than a superficial whitewash. Not satisfied either he or the information he held was secure, Ryan contacted newspaper columnist Jack Anderson, and television news reporter Daniel Schorr to document his evidence that Jonestown was a CIA operation. Later, posthumously, Congressman Ryan would be chastised for leaking government secrets to the press. Ryan then sealed a letter, detailing the CIA's sponsorship of Jonestown, along with instructions on what to do upon his death. The letter was addressed to Ryan's daughter Patricia, and entrusted to his attorney, Joe Holsinger. With as many insurance policies in place as Ryan could muster, he set out to die.

Ryan's party was forced to wait in Georgetown until Mark Lane arrived. Lane left the Assassinations Hearings and flew to Guyana to join the others. Permission was granted and the group boarded a plane bound for Jonestown. Bonnie Malmin and the Stoens cleverly decided to stay behind in Georgetown. On board the flight were Ryan, his assistant, Jackie Speier, Dick Dwyer, the Deputy Chief of Mission at the US Embassy (and a CIA operative), Neville Annibourne, an official of the Guyanese Ministry of Information (the CIA's counterpart), attorneys Mark Lane and Charles Garry, eight newsmen, Gordon Lindsay, and as many Concerned Relatives as there were remaining empty seats on the plane. Jones had hired Garry years earlier because he had a reputation for representing black radicals and Jones wanted to know everything he knew about the black revolutionary movement in the US.

They flew for about an hour over some of the most remote jungle in the world before the small dirt airstrip at Port Kaituma appeared below. As they disembarked, they were met by a group of armed temple guards, a minister of the Guyanese Regional Development, and "Corporal Rudder" who was introduced as the local chief of police. Rudder had no uniform or badge and his only claim to authority was the shotgun carried by his young assistant. The armed guards were probably part of the assault team sent in first to identify who was who and establish their targets for the next day's killings.

At first, Corporal Rudder announced that no one would be allowed to go to Jonestown. After a conference with Dwyer, it was agreed that Ryan, Speier, Dwyer, Lane, and Garry could go, but the reporters and Concerned Relatives could not and were sequestered on the hot, humid airstrip. The reporters sent a local into the village for two cases of cold Banks beer. They relaxed in the shade of a passenger shed, drinking beer and listening to Rudder's assistant tell tales of Jonestown escapees who reported brutal treatment in the encampment. He talked about strange nighttime activities at the airstrip that temple guards lit with flares for mysterious landings in the dark. The reporters were developing a relationship with the young constable who carried the shotgun that would be used to kill Congressman Ryan and three of their own.

In about two hours, the Jonestown farm tractor appeared in the clearing. A Caucasian woman standing behind a black driver announced, "Everyone who wants to come out to Jonestown can come, except Gordon Lindsay. The truck is coming." Lindsay did not appear disappointed at missing what he claimed was his only chance to see Jonestown. He boarded the twin engine Otter for the flight back to Georgetown where he set up a command center at the Pegasus Hotel, the only decent accommodations in the capital. As agreed, he phoned in his colleague's first reports. For the next few days, all reports regarding Jonestown came from Gordon Lindsay, simply because he had the only telephone. Lindsay never wrote a book or even an article about Jonestown, but there is not a single news report about the next few critical days that was not first filtered through him.

By the time the reporters arrived in Jonestown, it was dark and they were brought to the pavilion to reunite with Ryan and meet Jones. The entire community was gathered there to enjoy what has been described as a very delicious barbequed pork dinner. The only one who did not partake was Mark Lane, who chose instead the cough drops he had brought with him. This would later be used to discredit Lane who some claimed had prior knowledge that the dinner might have been poisoned. The truth is Jones had served pork to his Jewish attorney. To most of the residents and some of the news crew, this was a "condemned man's last meal." Immediately after dinner, the very professional and very loud "Jonestown Express" rock and roll band began the night's entertainment right in front of the visitors. Ryan managed to comment to some of the reporters that the residents appeared to be in a trace and "unnaturally animated." Jackie Speier said, "There is no question in my mind that mind control is being exercised here."

Ryan took the microphone to address the residents. "I can tell you right now that by the few conversations I have had with some of the folks here already this evening that there are some people who believe this is the best thing that ever happened in their whole lives." The crowd erupted in roaring applause that lasted for an incredible twenty minutes. When Ryan was finally free to speak, he joked that he wished they could all vote in his district. Jones yelled back, "They can, by absentee ballot." Ryan then got serious, telling the gathering, "I want to pull no punches. This is a Congressional inquiry."

The music stopped, the evening was over. Without so much as a word, the residents returned to their cabins. Ryan, Dwyer, Lane, and Garry were escorted to the East House, a cabin that just days earlier had been the home of Lisa Layton. Jones concluded a brief interview with the reporters by claiming there was a conspiracy to destroy the Peoples Temple. When asked who was plotting his demise, he said, "Who conspired to kill Martin Luther King and John Kennedy. Every agency of the US government is giving us a hard time." It was a simple diversion. Jones was planting seeds in the reporters' minds that he was paranoid, and persecuted by the US government, when in fact, he was a very sane, calculating employee of that same government. The reporters asked to sleep on the pavilion floor, but Jones insisted they return to Port Kaituma where he had arranged for their accommodations. They left disappointed at having learned so little. If they did not have a mouthful of barbeque, they had an earful of amplified music or roaring applause. There was no time for meaningful conversation and that was exactly what Jones intended. As they boarded the truck for Port Kaituma, Don Harris was handed a note that read, "Help us get out of Jonestown— Vern Gosney and Monica Bagby." The reporters and Concerned Relatives were taken to Mike's Disco and Rum House, a shack in Port Kaituma, stocked with rum and nothing else, not even a bathroom. They were told they could sleep on the floor.

The following morning, the temple truck returned two hours late to take them back to Jonestown where they got their first look at the community in the light of day. They were impressed with the well organized town, but the residents seemed rather bizarre. They were emotionless zombies, just walking through the day as if they weren't even there. A group of children played lethargically nearby as if they had been ordered to do so. Any time a reporter ventured off the tour he was met with, "Can I help you" and herded back in line. Ryan received more notes, mostly from Caucasians. In all, fifteen people wanted to leave Jonestown. Jones consulted with each of them, either to convince them to stay or to give them final instructions. Jones acted upset at the little more than one percent of his followers who wanted to leave, even though some claimed that they would return after visiting relatives in California. Jones grasped his heart, as if in pain, and asked his wife for "A pill," loud enough for the reporters to hear. They would later report that the paranoid cult leader had a drug habit, failing to realize that Jones was manipulating them. Their reports would later help justify what was going to happen next.

Ryan wanted to stay another night to document anyone else who wanted to leave, but this would upset Jones's schedule. Dick Dwyer had slipped away earlier to prepare the assassination team in Port Kaituma. Everything was in place and Jones would not allow Ryan to ruin his plans. Ryan needed to leave now. Jones's strong-arm man, Don Sly, approached Ryan from behind, grabbed him in a strangle hold, and put a knife to his throat. "I'm going to kill you, you mother fucker!" he shouted. Sly could have easily killed Ryan. He was a very burly man who had once trained for the Olympics, but this was not the time or the place. Lane and Garry wrestled the knife from Sly, but not before someone was cut. Ryan was spattered in blood and noticeably shaken. Ryan's party and the defectors ran for the truck but, at the last minute Larry Layton joined the group after huddling with Jones. There was a sense of relief as they drove away, relief that Ryan was not hurt and the defectors had gotten out alive, but everyone was nervous about Larry Layton who the residents claimed was too close to Jones to be a true defector. In an unusual show of compassion, Jones had given each of the defectors their passports and $5,000 cash for the passage home.

Ryan's party arrived at the airstrip to find three planes, the Otter from the day before, and a Cessna. Ryan had used Jonestown's radio to request additional transportation for the defectors. There was a third craft— a large military cargo plane parked perpendicular to the end of the runway, so all the windows on the right side had an unobstructed view of the entire airstrip. Next to the aircraft was a tent with about six armed soldiers, dressed in Guyanese Defense Forces uniforms, protecting what was reported as a "disabled plane."

Larry Layton immediately boarded the Cessna, hid a .38 caliber Smith and Wesson revolver, and exited to join the others who were milling about, deciding who would go on which plane and loading baggage. Dwyer told Ryan that it would be prudent for him to pat down all the passengers for concealed weapons to avert any possible problems. Just as soon as Ryan had searched all the passengers and told Dwyer that no one was armed, the Jonestown truck and farm tractor with trailer emerged from the jungle. The truck stopped, but the tractor approached Ryan's party. The tractor driver demanded to know who was leaving on which plane and the lack of any apparent reason for him knowing, struck fear in the group. Dick Dwyer, Corporal Rudder, and his assistant moved away to a vantage point on the edge of the airstrip just before the first gun shots were fired. Some of the assault team walked over to a group of local bystanders and pushed them out of the way, while three assassins walked forward carrying a military issued M-16 assault rifles. They first sprayed Ryan's party with gunfire from left to right, aiming well below the waist and shooting out the tires of one of the planes. Jonestown defector Patty Parks was killed in this first assault, but only because she was bent down over her luggage at the time. Her death appears to have been an accident. This first volley was clearly not meant to kill, only to wound. Everyone hit the ground, some because they were wounded, the rest because they were frightened. Everyone, that is except Dick Dwyer, Corporal Rudder, and his shotgun toting assistant who stood off to one side. Larry Layton had scrambled back into the Cessna, retrieved the revolver, and shot and wounded defectors Vern Gosney and Monica Bagby. He fired at the pilot, but missed. He then tried to shoot defector Dale Parks. There was gun fire, but no bullet, as if the gun had been loaded with a blank. Parks wrestled the gun from Layton as the second assault began. The leader of the assassination team approached Dwyer, Corporal Rudder, and his assistant, who were standing off to one side, where they had been since just before the shooting began. Meanwhile, reporter Ron Javers was begging the Guyanese soldiers for help, but they refused, saying, "These are Americans killing Americans and none of our business." Rudder's assistant handed his shotgun to Dwyer, who handed it to the assassin who used it to shoot Congressman Ryan four times in the head. He fatally shot cameramen Bob Brown and Greg Robinson. He then turned his weapon on Don Harris and blew his head off. Harris was a talented investigator with two areas of expertise— the assassination of Martin Luther King and the CIA's connections to Howard Hughes. Don Harris was as much of a target at the airstrip as was Congressman Ryan.

The assassination team retreated back into the jungle. Dead were Congressman Ryan, Don Harris, Patty Parks, and cameramen Bob Brown and Greg Robinson, who bravely filmed their own murders. In all, five were dead, five seriously wounded, and five slightly wounded, though it is a stretch to call Charles Krause's injuries a wound. He suffered a scratch on his leg while trying to hide in the baggage compartment of the Cessna. Dwyer immediately took charge. Parks brought him Layton's gun. Dwyer claimed to have been grazed by a bullet in his buttocks, but this was just good theater; he did not seek any medical treatment and no one was about to verify his alleged wound. Dwyer ordered the seriously wounded to be carried on makeshift bedspring litters to the soldiers who agreed to house them for the night, not in the disabled plane, but in their tent. The dead were left on the airstrip overnight, but Dwyer needed everyone else to leave. He shouted, "They're coming back! They're coming back!" which was enough of a threat to send the survivors into the bush for cover. While the reporters hid in the jungle, Dwyer ordered the two pilots to fly the last operative plane back to Georgetown with only Monica Bagby on board even though there were several empty seats. Dwyer did not want the reporters communicating with the outside world; that was Gordon Lindsay's job; nor did he have the humanity to send the seriously wounded back for medical care. It was getting dark and Dwyer confiscated the only flashlight in the group. He rounded up the terrorized survivors and brought them back to Mike's Disco and Rum Bar for another night of hard drinking.

Dwyer spent the evening between the rum bar, the airstrip, and Jonestown, being away from each location for hours at a time. Alone, he was free to rummage through the pockets and possessions of the dead to confiscate anything incriminating about Jonestown, including Ryan's briefcase containing all of his notes and audio recordings of the trip. The FBI searched for the briefcase for over a week, but failed to locate it. Suddenly, it reappeared, delivered to the doorstep of Joe Holsinger back in California. The lock had been broken and anything of importance had been removed. All that remained were blank cassette tapes, stationary, a dime, a comb and two business cards.

Ryan's assassination at the airstrip leaves many unanswered questions. The truck and the tractor, pulling the trailer returned too soon to have returned to Jonestown, so the assault team had to be hiding in the jungle. Why did they rely on Corporal Rudder's shotgun and not bring their own? How did they know it would not be used against them? Who was Rudder's assistant who provided the murder weapon? No one knows because, as difficult as it is to believe, no one has ever asked. Finally, there remains the definitive question, who fired the gun that killed the congressman? Thirty-five years later, we still do not know who killed Ryan.

Jonestown was a tight-knit group, that had lived together for many months. If the assassin was a temple guard, certainly one of the defectors at the airstrip would have recognized him, but no one did.

Back in Jonestown, about a dozen nurses and Dr. Schacht mixed the fifteen gallon vat of potassium cyanide, grape Flavor-Aid and liquid tranquilizers Valium and Darvon. The staff filled hypodermic needles, squeeze bottles, and hundreds of paper cups with the poison. Jones took the microphone, switched on a tape recorder, and ordered everyone to the pavilion— the White Night was about to begin. "Take Dwyer to the East House. No, not Ujara! I said, take Dwyer to the East House," Jones repeated, just to document Dwyer's presence at the massacre, whether he was actually there or not. Jones ordered attorneys Lane and Garry to the East House, and to be certain they complied, he had Don Sly escort them, the same man who had assaulted Ryan earlier that day.

As a footnote to Don Sly, he was also known as "Ujara" which is very unsettling. In the CIA's **MK ULTRA** quest to induce multiple personalities, they often labeled the subject's alternate personality with obscure African names. Calling his name could trigger the change and create the assassin, so they had to be careful not to name him anything that might come up in idle conversation.

Over the PA, Jones shouted:

"The Congressman is Dead! The Congressman is Dead!
Come to the pavilion. What a legacy! What a legacy! It's
time to pass over. This isn't just a suicide. It's a revolutionary

suicide. Come my children before the CIA parachutes in here to castrate, rape, and kill."

Jones had learned from Mengele that quiet, reflective music helped sooth the nerves of those who were about to die. Mengele had a string quartet play outside the gas chambers. Jones selected two melacholy songs by singer/song writer, Marvin Gaye to play in rotation over the public address system. The first was *"Mercy, Mercy Me,"* a song about how human overpopulation has taxed the earth's resources. The second was *"What's Going On,"* that laments war, protest and man's intolerance of his fellow man. The residents recognized these popular songs, but it is doubtful that anyone, except Jones, recognized their significance to the event taking place. During the song's repetitions on the PA, Jones gave words of encouragement:

> "Please get the medication before it's too late.
> The GDF [Guyanese Defense Force] will be
> here ... don't be afraid to die ... It's all over ...
> The Congressman is dead ... How many are
> dead? It isn't painful, just a little bitter tasting."

The first to die in Jonestown were the babes-in-arms. Jones ordered mothers to bring their youngest up to the vat first. Nurses squirted poison into the baby's mouths, but not the mothers. Annie Moore selected the proper colored marker from a box and put an "X" on the mother's right hand to designate her willingness to kill her child and then sent them off to witness their babies die in her arms. The mother's turn would come later. Jones had promised his CIA sponsors that he could get black people to kill themselves and this is not an easy task as, statistically, blacks are the least likely group to commit suicide. Jones was using every trick to improve those odds. Obviously, the infants had not reached the age of reason and were not a part of the experiment. Once the mothers had killed their babies, there was little left for them to live for and they were more open to committing suicide themselves.

The next to die were the older children who had at least some reasoning. Their willingness and that of the parents was noted with the proper colored marker on their right hands. The adults were next. Many drank the poison, but many refused and were forcibly injected. Again, each was marked with the appropriate colored marker to record their voluntary participation or lack there of. Despite Jones's assurances that it was not painful, those towards the back of the line could hear the screams of those in the front. Death from cyanide poisoning takes a few minutes and is extremely excruciating. Victims foam at the mouth and suffer wild, uncontrollable convulsions. Some die with their back arched and just their forehead and the heels of their feet touching the ground. With hundreds flailing on the ground, the scene must have been horrific.

Temple guards, armed with automatic weapons, hunting bows and crossbows, formed two concentric circles around the pavilion. Jones referred to the later as his, "Silent Weapons Squad." The use of crossbows may seem out of place, but they served a purpose. Jones realized that many would run and needed to be stopped, but he did not want the sound of gun fire on the PA's tape recorder that he intended to leave as an official historic record. In one post-Jonestown news video there can be clearly seen a spent arrow lodged in a trash receptacle. It was tipped, not with a target point, but a razor-sharp, four sided hunting point designed to kill. The runners were shot, wrestled to the ground and injected in the back with a hypodermic filled with cyanide. Even Jonestown's guard dogs and their chimpanzee mascot, Mr. Muggs, were killed.

From time to time, Jones left the pavilion for various errands. One time he radioed the temple's Georgetown administrative offices to instruct them to begin their own White Night. When asked, "How?" Jones spelled out "K-N-I-F-E". Temple aide, Sharon Amos and her three children died from having their throats slit with a large kitchen knife. The official report claims it was a murder/suicide, but many believe that it was just murder committed by long-time temple aide, Charles Beikman, who witnessed the deaths, but survived uninjured. Beikman was a Caucasian, ex-Marine who had been with Jones since the late 1950s. He managed the temple's thrift store in Kumaka, a village in Northern Guyana. As further evidence of premeditation, the store went out of business just one week before the massacre.

Jones then radioed temple headquarters in San Francisco with a simple, three word order, "Shred everything now". It was about 2 p.m., San Francisco time, and the temple staff worked tirelessly for the next 24 hours shredding every piece of paper in the building. When the news of Jonestown's demise first reached San Francisco the next day, there was not a single piece of printed evidence left to support that the Peoples Temple had ever existed.

Several people were allowed to leave the White Night. Attorneys Lane and Garry were set free to make their way on foot, in the dark, back to Port Kaituma where, the next morning they were reunited with the airstrip survivors. Jonestown guards like former Special Forces soldier Odell Rhodes, were also allowed to leave as was Stanley Clayton and Tim Carter. Rhodes and Carter would play significant roles.

Ex-marine and Jonestown guard Tim Carter contributed more to the Jonestown project in the aftermath than he did while it occurred. For the next thirty-five years, Carter was always featured in television documentaries. Carter, along with Deborah Layton, molded the public's opinion of Jones. While Layton told America that Jones was paranoid and insane, Carter emphasized his alleged drug dependency. Together, they double teamed the American conscience. Just before the White Night, Carter was back in California, where, alone with Deborah Layton, he joined the Concerned Relatives to monitor Congressman Ryan's trip plans. Despite what appeared to be an obvious transgression and defection, Jones accepted him back into Jonestown just prior to the event. According to Carter, he tried to escape the final carnage by asking Jones if he could help chase down some of the runners who had fled into the jungle. All reports claim that Jones gave him a suitcase full of money with instructions to give it to the Russian Embassy in Georgetown to "further the socialist cause" but after that, reports vary so much in detail as to question what really happened. Carter set out on foot in the dark to either Port Kaituma where he was arrested or to Matthew's Ridge where he followed the train tracks back to Georgetown. All accounts claim the money was too heavy to carry so Carter either buried it or discarded it by the wayside. Depending on who you choose to believe, the cash entrusted to Carter was somewhere between 30 and 750 thousand dollars but the discrepancies are academic because none of it ever reached the Russian Embassy. It was just another one of Jones's disinformation ploys. All agree that three days later, Carter was under arrest in Georgetown but eventually set free and returned to the US to accept a position as a police officer in Hawaii. He had "escaped" Jonestown, but not the experiment as, according to him, today he is HIV positive. The problem with this scenario is that Carter was back in Jonestown the next morning, helping to identify bodies. If he walked to Matthews Ridge he would have been on a direct collision course with the first responders from Georgetown. The first responders including CIA operative Dan Webber, Guyana's First Lady, Viola Burnham, Chief Coroner Dr. Mootoo, his assistants, and a company of Guyanese Defense Forces troops had taken a train to Matthews Ridge. In all probability, Carter's real task was to meet them in Matthews Ridge and guide them back to Jonestown. The suitcase full of money has never been accounted for.

The first responders arrived in Jonestown the morning after. Of this we are certain, but, what we do not know is when their preparations began. They had to walk twenty miles from Matthews Ridge after a three-hour train trip, but there had not been train service to Matthews Ridge for years, ever since Burnham had nationalized US owned bauxite mines located there. First, they needed to arrange for a train and crew. Then, they had to call up and supply the troops. Working backwards from their morning after arrival, timing would dictate that they would have had to start planning prior to even Ryan's arrival in Guyana. This may be an indication that the Guyanese government, or more specifically, the CIA in Georgetown, knew in advance that Ryan would be killed and Jonestown would self-destruct.

Jonestown security guards were mostly former US Marines and Army Special Forces, probably left over from the mercenary trainers in the Shalom Project. It would require several additional books to present a detailed history of all of them. The best that can be accomplished here is a brief history of one prime example. Odell Rhodes was born to a poor black family in Detroit. At age seventeen, he quit school and joined the army. After three tours in Korea and a reenlistment, he was sent to Fort Carson, Colorado and assigned to a program conceived by President Kennedy and Defense Secretary Robert McNamara. It was intended to be the army's elite commando fighting force— the "Special Forces" as it was named. At the first graduation ceremonies, with Kennedy and McNamara in the reviewing stands, it was Odell Rhodes who was chosen to carry the company's colors. He was not the cream of the army's crop. He was the cream of the cream of the army's crop. According to Rhodes's autobiography, soon afterwards, he was falsely charged with a minor infraction, court-martialed, dishonorably discharged, and incarcerated in Leavenworth Prison, but none of this makes any sense because, according to Rhodes, he was then released from prison, his discharge was rescinded, and he was reassigned to the army's chemical arsenal at Fort McClellan, Alabama. Both Leavenworth Prison and Fort McClellan were sites of CIA **MK ULTRA** experiments. After jungle combat training, Rhodes was sent to Vietnam and then back to Korea. Eventually, he was honorably discharged in Washington, D.C. in 1968. He returned to Detroit. As the cover story goes, Jim Jones was taking his followers on a cross country bus tour when they found Rhodes struggling on the streets of Detroit as a heroin addict. Jones took him in, brought him back to California, and gave him a job supervising one of the temple's foster care homes. In the final analysis, Rhodes was one of only a few black people in the temple's hierarchy.

The next day, the wounded at the airstrip, Vern Gosney, Anthony Kataris, Beverly Oliver and Howard Oliver were evacuated by helicopter to Puerto Rico for medical treatment. All survived. Gosney went on to become a police officer in Hawaii, as did Tim Carter, which leads one to question whether their service in Jonestown was rewarded with a good job in paradise.

Very early the next morning, Congressman Ryan's attorney Joe Holsinger received a phone call from the State Department informing him that his long time friend had been murdered. When Holsinger asked how they knew, they responded that they had a CIA agent at the airstrip who had used the radio in Jonestown to broadcast the message over a secret CIA frequency. Actually, it was a "flash message"— a top secret means of communicating very brief messages to CIA headquarters that is usually reserved for emergencies. The logical sender was Dick Dwyer, who was listed in the *Whose Who in the CIA,* but there were so many CIA assets involved that it is difficult to identify the caller. Back at the US Embassy in Georgetown was Ambassador John Burke, who had worked for the CIA since 1963 and partnered with Dwyer in Bangkok, Thailand during the Vietnam War. Also at the embassy was Chief Consular Officer Richard McCoy, a military intelligence asset who was very close to Jones and on loan to the embassy from the Defense Department. Another previously identified CIA agent, Dan Webber, was the first to arrive at the scene in Jonestown the next morning. After all the smoke had cleared, the surviving Jonestown defectors were represented by attorney Joseph Blatchford who graciously offered his services pro bono, but failed to disclose that he had previously been named in a scandal involving the CIA's infiltration of the Peace Corp. In addition to the CIA operatives on site, there were the "eyes and ears only" agency technicians inside the so-called "disabled" military cargo plane who had filmed the entire assassination. But, in the end, the flash message that Ryan and the residents of Jonestown were all dead was sent hours before any outsiders entered Jonestown. The CIA had to be on site when it all went down.

The first outsiders to view the carnage arrived the next morning to find all the bodies face down in nice, neat rows, head-to-head, toe-to toe, all organized by family for easy identification. Obviously, a group of residents had survived. It had to be a 'group' because it would have taken a considerable labor force to drag all those bodies into position and they had to be 'residents' because the people who did this needed to know the victims personally in order to group them by family. Logically, the survivors would have been the guards, commanded by Jones. A person looking like Jones was found dead of a gunshot wound to the head next to Jones's throne. Despite the fact that this was a dangerous place, with mass murders and suicides, Prime Minister Forbes Burnham sent his wife, Viola, in charge of the first responders. She headed a group of CIA operatives, Guyanese Defense Forces troops, the country's Chief Medical Examiner Dr. C. Leslie Mootoo, and a few of his assistants. They ransacked Jonestown looking for anything of value. Reportedly, the First Lady left with a million dollars in cash. Dr. Mootoo remained to work thirty-two straight hours to examine at least some of the bodies before he ran out of energy and supplies. He petitioned the US government for help, but was denied. He conducted autopsies and found that some had cyanide and Valium in their stomach contents and some just in their bloodstream. Of those he examined, he determined that at least "eighty-three people had been injected with cyanide" and obviously murdered. They were particularly interested in the body of young Nawab Laurence. Dr. Mootoo's assistant recognized the eleven-year-old boy from when he passed through Guyana customs. Laurence had been born a heroin addict in California; one of many in Jonestown.

Washington was slow to react. The State Department recommended that Guyana dig a pit and bulldoze the bodies into a mass grave. San Francisco Mayor George Moscone strongly objected and telegrammed President Carter to say,

> "I respectfully request that you use your
> authority to underwrite the cost of
> bringing back those whose next of kin
> request that they be returned and
> who otherwise do not have the means
> to do so."

To President Carter, this seemed to be a compassionate request, and, besides, the government could always recoup the expense by seizing temple assets. To the rather touchy CIA this looked like a veiled threat, implying US government responsibly for the deaths. Moscone presented a problem, but only for a little more than a week until they killed him too.

There was really no investigation into the deaths, either at the airstrip or in Jonestown. The CIA was there, but they were not about to investigate themselves. The Guyana government did not care, like the soldiers at the airstrip said, "These were Americans killing Americans and none of their business." Guyana **did** do one thing for their CIA sponsors, they forbid the FBI from entering their country. There was one official investigation conducted by three staff members of the House Foreign Affairs Committee who relied on interviews with State Department officials, CIA personnel, and former Temple members. The Assassination of Representative Leo J. Ryan and the Jonestown, Guyana Tragedy (House Committee on Foreign Affairs—Document #96-223, 96th Congress) was released on May 15th, 1979. The report is riddled with errors, but at times is surprisingly accurate. It reads:

> "Who and what was Jim Jones? We believe it is accurate to say he was charismatic in some respects: in fact, he was especially adroit in the area of human psychology. As we have studied him and interviewed those who knew him well and come under his influence, we have concluded that he was first and foremost a master of mind control."

So much for the truth. The committee's findings did present several factors indicating a conspiracy to kill Ryan:

> -The arrival of the cyanide, two days before Ryan's visit.
> -The planting of a temple spy ,Tim Carter, in the Concerned Relatives group to monitor Ryan's trip plans.
> -The start of the White Night some twenty minutes prior to the assault team's return to Jonestown.
> -Reports that Jones implied Ryan would be killed several days before he arrived.

Though the committee could not avoid reporting such hard evidence, they dismissed the entire concept of a conspiracy with the following preamble:

> "The possibility of any prior conspiracy tends to be diminished by the fact that Gordon Lindsay, a reporter whom  Mr. Jones regarded as an arch enemy of Peoples Temple, was not allowed to enter Jonestown with the Ryan party."

Gordon Lindsay never did anything to hurt Jones, the Peoples Temple, or Jonestown. He did not file a complaint, write a book or an exposé or even a magazine article. The only reason that the congressional committee dismissed the conspiracy theory was that they believed Lindsay was an enemy because Jones had said so and therein lies the problem. They agree that Jones was a master of mind control, but apparently not of their minds, only other peoples'.

The US government did not care about the dead, but they certainly cared about any information that could link them to the carnage. President Carter's National Security Adviser Zbigniew Brezezinski, ordered that all the bodies be searched for any "political papers." Brezezinski passed his orders onto Robert Pastor, who passed them on to Lt. Col. Gordon Sumner, whose troops stripped the bodies of all identification and papers. Pastor would later be promoted deputy director of the CIA. None of the evidence collected at Jonestown or at the airstrip has ever surfaced. When Lt. Sumner arrived, he found that many of the bodies had identification tags attached to their right hands, obviously placed there by Jones's guards for the final documentation of the experiments. The tags are clearly visible in the **Newsweek** cover aerial photo, but were removed by Lt. Col. Sumner's men. Half of the victims would never be identified.

The first responders ransacked Jones's cabin. His large library was spread out on the front yard. As expected, half the books were on Nazi Germany and half were on techniques of mind control. They were probably looking for the extensive medical records that had been meticulously kept on every resident for over a year. The records contained the results of both experiments. What was the best drug cocktail to control blacks and how was AIDS transmitted? These answers and the medical records were never found or reported to have been found.

San Francisco newspaper headlines first reported that 400 were dead. Days later, the headlines read 780 dead. Days later they reported the final death toll as 903. The only explanation given for the ascending body count was that, as bodies were removed, more bodies were discovered hidden underneath. That would mean that initially 400 bodies covered 503 others, which is highly unlikely.

There is another explanation for the ascending body count. Perhaps only 400 people killed themselves and the remaining 503 fled into the jungle. This would not be a bad percentage for Jones's experiment, but it presented a problem. The runners could not be allowed to survive because many of them were HIV-positive and would pinpoint the origin of the epidemic. Coincidentally, (and there is no such thing as coincidence) there were 300 US

Special Forces Troops and 600 British Black Watch Commandoes on "training maneuvers" in the immediate vicinity at the time. It is possible that they rounded up the survivors, injected them with cyanide, and dragged their bodies back to Jonestown to be placed in the neat rows that they were found. When the body count fell short, the US Army's Special Forces sent helicopter gun ships over the surrounding jungle, announcing over loudspeakers that it was safe to return to Jonestown. They later claimed that this was a futile exercise when the missing victims were found under the bodies of the others.

Lt. Col. James "Bo" Gritz was the most decorated solider in the Vietnam War and the officer in charge of all US Special Forces in Latin America. His heroism and military record were the inspiration for the movie character "Rambo," He was in Guyana with his troops at the time, but did not go into Jonestown. A Green Beret commander took some of his men in, but not Gritz, who later recounted in his autobiography that the operation was "top secret, compartmentalized, on a need to know basis" and he did not need to know. Gritz talked with several of his men as they returned and saw in their eyes a look he had not seen since the Vietnam War when soldiers returned from an atrocity. One very angry soldier, SFC Sergeant Inman, told Gritz he was going to write a book, entitled, 'All The Niggers Are Dead.' When he asked the soldier, "Why so offensive a title?", he responded, "It doesn't make a difference what your color, your creed or your sex, when you allow yourself to be treated the way they were, that's what you are; you're a nigger and nothing else."

There is another peculiarity about the body count—there are over 150 people still missing. 1,200 US citizens presented their passports to Guyana customs with the stated intention of relocating to Jonestown. Thirty-three children were born in the community, so the total number should be 1,233, but there were subtractions. A few weeks before Jonestown, there was the exodus of top aides like Deborah Layton, Terri Buford, Paula Adams, Bonnie Malmin, and the Stoens. There was another exodus a few days before by Lisa Layton, the Baldwins, and Phil Blakey. Then there were the defectors who survived the airstrip, like Larry Layton, Vern Gosney, Monica Bagby, and Dale Parks. Jones's sons, both natural and adopted, were all conveniently in Georgetown at the time to play an exhibition basketball game. Guards like Tim Carter, Odell Rhodes, Stanley Clayton, Tom Kice, Sr., Albert Touchette, Joe Wilson, and Charles Beikman were also allowed to survive. Then there was Hyacinth Thrash, an elderly resident who retired to her cabin early and slept through the entire White Night. One unconfirmed report claims that

Hyacinth Thrash was actually Lisa Layton in disguise. A Venezuelan Air Force pilot patrolling the border reported that forty heavily armed Americans crossed over into Venezuela the morning after Jonestown. A head count of every possible person in Jonestown, less every possible person who could have left, adds up to over 150 people short. Since none of the missing 150 have ever resurfaced in Guyana or the United States, in all probability, they died in Jonestown prior to the White Night. These poor souls may have been the first victims of AIDS.

# T H I R T E E N

## ESCAPE AND DEPLOYMENT

*"All is a riddle and the key to a riddle is another riddle."*

**—Ralph Waldo Emerson.**

In early November, 1978, two weeks before the White Night, Jones summoned several of his young homosexual male followers to a private meeting. There were many homosexual men in Jonestown, just as there had been in San Francisco, from where they were recruited, but these were special. Jones had hand picked them from the start. Since sex in Jonestown, including homosexual sex, was prohibited without Jones's permission and often command, it was easy to document the transmission of the HIV virus through the community. Jones held this group until the very end when he ordered them to have sex with other residents whose medical records indicated they had the virus. Members of this group were infected so recently that they did not yet exhibit any symptoms. As a reward for their hard work, Jones gave each a large sum of cash and the opportunity for an all expense paid vacation. They would board the *Albatross* in Port Kaituma for a voyage to Port-au-Prince, Haiti, where they could stay for as long as they wanted. Jones encouraged them to enjoy themselves and spend their reward money in the many homosexual brothels in the suburb of Carrefour. Carrefour had an international reputation for catering to the gay tourist trade. It was the preferred winter vacation destination for young gay men from Manhattan. The season begins in December with the first snowfall in New York City, but it does not peak until February or early March during Carnival. Jones's task force unknowingly infected Haitian prostitutes who, in turn, infected the gay US sex tourists, who brought the virus back to the United States. Since Jones was not actually operating on US soil, his actions under the rules of the CIA might have been considered "legal". Some say that "AIDS Patient Zero" was a French airline steward whose good looks, insatiable sexual appetite, and world travel, fueled the spread of the disease. Port-au-Prince was a frequent destination for this gay Frenchman.

Jones sent his gay task force to Haiti in early November, 1978. Jonestown self-destructed two weeks later. The first reported cases of GRID or Gay-Related Immune Deficiency (known today as AIDS), was traced back to Haiti in December, 1978. The first cases in the United States were reported in New York City gays in January, 1979. November, December, January, 1,2,3. Timing is everything.

With all of his long-term planning, one might think that Jones would have been concerned with his own ultimate survival, and he was. Even in the earliest rehearsals of the White Night, the plan was always for Jones to survive. In the end, the FBI positively identified the body of "Jim Jones," but the truth is, the real Jim Jones got away clean and this is how he did it.

Jones purchased yet another former Jewish Synagogue, this time in Los Angeles, far away from watchful eyes in San Francisco. He bussed his congregation to L.A. once a week for services. He never had much success recruiting followers in L.A., but what he did have was an escape plan. In November of 1973, five years before the final "White Night", Jones secured an agreement with the government of Guyana to lease over 4,000 acres of jungle that would become Jonestown. He had opened a door and, in that same month, he devised a plan to close it.

It started at an L.A. service in which he announced, "I have had a revelation that something strange might happen tonight. No matter what happens, I don't want anyone to call an ambulance." An elderly black parishioner named Pinky, collapsed at the back of the congregation. Jones's wife, Marceline, defied her husband's order and phoned for help. Marceline, their adopted son, Jimmy, and temple guard, Cleveland Jackson, carried Pinky on a stretcher out to an adjoining alley to an awaiting ambulance, where they immediately started a fist fight with the Emergency Medical Technicians, one of whom broke away to radio the police. Twelve uniformed officers and a swat team helicopter responded. Jones's son punched an officer and broke his nose. Marceline Jones began screaming, ranting and raving in a technique of intimidation the Caucasian temple aides called "crazy niggering". Marceline, her son, and the guard were taken into custody to the Ramparts Police Station. In all the confusion, other temple guards brought Pinky back inside. Jones left the services, but sent a surrogate to the Ramparts Station where he was so abusive to the police that they locked him in the cell with the others. Marceline and the man she claimed was her husband were released without being charged. A few days later, the others were released as well. This first attempt to have his surrogate arrested had failed, but Jones continued to try.

He embarked on a vicious letter writing campaign demanding an apology from the LAPD. He was obviously trying to antagonize the police, and by casting mainly his family members, he showed the importance of this theatrical production and the venue, far away from the scrutiny of his home base in San Francisco, was of equal importance.

Temple members were forbidden to spend money on movie tickets, but, on his next weekly visit to L.A. Jones broke his own rules, and took his adopted son to see a movie at the nearby Westlake Theater. Afterwards, Jones claimed his son was harassed by an undercover vice squad officer. His set-up was complete.

Jones was a dangerous man, often in dangerous situations. It has been widely reported that he employed doubles to impersonate him. His followers called them "look-alikes". Two of his aides, Rheaviana Beam and Rose Shelton, carried the suitcase that contained the wigs and makeup to transform Wayne Pietila, Harold Cordell, Mike Prokes, and at least one other into clones of Jones. The deceit was easy. Jones himself was very "made up". He wore make up, dyed his hair jet black, and, day or night, he was never seen without his trademark CIA aviator-type sunglasses. No one knew what he really looked like. They did not have to make the doubles look like Jones, they only needed to make Jones and the doubles look like the same person. It was easy.

On December 13, 1973, Jones sent a "look-alike" to the Westlake Theater for what the double thought was an attempt to embarrass the vice squad officer, and the police in general, in order to avenge the incidents with Pinky and Jones's son. Totally out of character, Jones's double entered the theater alone and in street clothes. The real Jim Jones was never seen without his accompanying body guards. The double approached Officer A. L. Kagele in the men's room and, according to the arresting officer's report:

"Officer entered the rest room, and within a minute officer heard the rest room door open and observed the defendant. Officer observed the defendant's right arm moving, and at this point the defendant turned to the officer. Officer observed the defendant's penis to be erect, and the defendant, with his right hand was masturbating and showing his penis to the officer. The defendant then walked toward the officer with his erect penis in his hand. Officer exited the rest room and signaled his partner of the violation."

At 4 p.m., Officer A.L. Kagele and Officer Lloyd Frost arrested the defendant for "lewd conduct". He was taken into custody to the Ramparts Police Station where this "look-alike" was booked, photographed, and fingerprinted as "James Warren Jones". Tim Stoen posted the $500 bail and proceeded to enlist the help of everyone he knew in California law, including the State Attorney General. At the trial, Judge Clarence A. Stromwell dismissed the case "in the furtherance of justice" because "the defendant stipulated as to probable cause." No reason was ever given as required by law. Six weeks later, in the privacy of his chambers, and not the courtroom, the judge ordered the arrest and court records "sealed and destroyed" but somehow they survived. Tim Stoen made certain, by first consulting with Mike Franchetti, later the chief assistant to the attorney general of California, because, as Franchetti later recalled, "I was an expert in records law and how they were sealed." Neither the arrest nor trial were reported in the news. The censorship was so air tight that Jones was included in the list of "The 100 Outstanding Clergymen in America" immediately following the incident. A few months later, the **Los Angeles Herald Examiner** awarded Jones the "Humanitarian of the Year" award. Just before the White Night, Tim Stoen was working with the Concerned Relatives to convince Ryan to investigate Jonestown. He prepared a legal motion to have Jones's arrest records released to the public, which eventually they were four months **after** the White Night, but what Stoen was really interested in was the disclosure proceedings scheduled **before** the White Night, in which the L.A. courts revealed that they still possessed the files.

All of the Concerned Relatives who accompanied Ryan said that Jones did not look like the Jones they remembered from just a year and a half earlier. He was heavier and his facial features were different. Reporter Ron Javers later recalled that his first impression of Jones was that he was "powdered and perfumed." Reporter Charles Krause had another curiosity, as he later reported in his book on Jonestown:

> "I sat beside him (Jones) and watched him closely as he talked. Grace Stoen had told me that he used an eyebrow pencil to give an appearance of thickness to his sideburns. I was curious about that and, after looking at him for awhile, decided she was right."

Jones was holding Grace Stoen's son, John-John in Jonestown, against her will along with a thousand other Americans in a hell hole of a concentration camp of international, historic proportions and she was concerned with Jones's use of an eyebrow pencil on his sideburns? The truth is Grace Stoen was preparing the press for a cosmetic Jones who, in turn, prepared the world for a cosmetic corpse. Decades later, one of Jones's female aides stepped forward with a story that the corpse identified as Jones could not be him because Jones had a tattoo on his chest that was not in the photograph of the corpse, but since no one else has stepped forward who had seen Jones's chest in life and in death, her allegations can not be confirmed.

All the test persons in Jonestown were dead, and the guards shouted "Hip, Hip Hooray!" The unwitting double was seated in Jones's throne in the pavilion and shot behind the left ear, consistent with the suicide of a left-handed person, but Jones was right handed. The gun was found several yards away and someone had rested the head of the corpse on a pillow. The US State Department first asked Guyana to bulldoze a pit and bury the bodies in Jonestown, but San Francisco Mayor George Moscone convinced President Carter to use his authority to override the State Department and underwrite the expense of returning the dead to the US and their families. The corpses were placed, not in body bags, but in special hermetically-sealed aluminum coffins that the military designed for victims of biological warfare, or outbreaks of a communicable plague. The coffins were shipped to the military mortuary at Dover Air Force Base in Delaware. Chief Undertaker, Charles Carson, was in charge of the postmortem investigation that was universally condemned by the medical profession as, "inept, incompetent, and embarrassing." Carson destroyed all evidence by first draining the corpses of bodily fluids. No fluids or tissue samples were preserved for analysis. He was allowed to conduct only seven autopsies: Jim Jones, Larry Schacht, Marie Katsaris and four others of the FBI's choosing. The seven autopsies were performed, but only after the bodies had been embalmed. Dr. Rudiger Breitenecker, who assisted in the autopsies, later claimed that there was "a series of errors," He said, "We shudder at the degree of ineptness." The forensic pathologist and medical examiners trade magazine, **Lab World** published an article entitled, "Guyana: Autopsy of Disbelief" in which was written:

"The contradictions, inconsistencies, and questionable truths related through these interviews leave many unanswered questions. In fact the entire episode suggests government mismanagement or a cover up of the true facts...It is regrettable that professional medical personnel failed to do what the newest member—fresh from college—of a clinical medical laboratory would have known to do."

The President of the National Association of Medical Examiners, Dr. Sturmer, sent a harsh, open letter to the army, protesting the examinations that he characterized as " badly botched", as well as the illegal cremation of some bodies. There was no cause of death listed, no identification of the bodies, and no certificates of death issued. Even the prestigious **New England Journal of Medicine** raised objections. Realize, these were not radicals or conspiracy theorist. These are eminent doctors who claimed that there was a government cover-up. Most of the bodies were shipped to Oakland, where they were buried in a common grave.

The initial examinations of the corpses had been done by Guyana's Chief Medical Examiner, Dr. C. Leslie Mootoo, who found that many died from being needled in the back with cyanide. Dr. Mootoo sent his findings to the US Embassy in Georgetown, but they neglected to forward them on to Dr. Carson, who appears to have been instructed to destroy all evidence and touch nothing.

Indicative of the inept handling of the bodies was an episode that occurred seven years later in the southern California town of Carson. The manager of a Storage-R-Us facility broke into a self storage unit after the mortuary that had rented it failed to pay the bill. He called the authorities when he discovered three aluminum coffins inside. Based on the unusual coffins and the markings on the outside, the authorities determined that the occupants were victims from Jonestown. They never released their identities, but since half of the dead were never identified, in all probability, they did not know. This was seven years after the fact and these three victims had not been buried. No explanation has ever been given as to how or why the corpses made the additional 500 mile trip from Oakland to Carson. Eventually, the coffins were unlocked, unsealed, and opened to reveal a macabre surprise worthy of a horror movie. Inside two of them were two additional bodies. One was never identified, the other was an army veteran named Faustino Dominguez, who died in July of 1982. There is no indication that Dominguez had anything to do with Jonestown, but this story is so bizarre that nothing is out of the realm of possibility. The mortuary owner would eventually be convicted of only a misdemeanor violation of the state health code.

CIA agents are not allowed to lie; it is bad trade craft. If they are caught in a lie, it could jeopardize the entire operation. When confronted with a difficult question, they are instructed to be vague, hence the familiar response, "I can neither confirm, nor deny the allegation." The morning after the White Night, Dick Dwyer was asked to identify Jones's body. Despite the fact that Dwyer had been with Jones and Ryan the day before and may have returned to Jones later that evening, the next day he would not say yes or no. Dwyer would only say that he was "awfully certain" that the corpse was Jones. His ambiguity speaks volumes. The corpse was left to rot in the jungle heat for four days before being shipped to Delaware for identification. Ten FBI fingerprint experts surgically removed the fingertips, placed them over their own gloved fingers and inked prints. According to FBI Director, William Webster in a statement to the **San Francisco Chronicle**:

> "The identification of the preacher's remains was made soon after (arrival) by a team of ten FBI fingerprint specialists who compared Los Angeles Police Department records of Jones's prints with ones taken from his body, Webster said."

Ten fingerprint experts were needed? Why so many? One for each finger? Or was the government just trying to give the impression they were being thorough? At that time, the FBI was already in possession of testimony from temple members that Jones used "look-a-likes" and had a plan to escape Jonestown via a flight from Venezuela to Africa. The so-called fingerprint experts were so intent on the details of lines and patterns under their microscopes that they failed to see the big picture. Yes, the fingerprints matched, but they did not match Jim Jones's. They matched the double that he had sent on a bizarre mission to the Westlake Theater.

Jones's wife, Marceline, really did die in Jonestown. Her body was positively identified at the Dover Air Force Base Mortuary by her parents, the Baldwins, and as the last surviving next of kin, they requested that "Jim" and Marceline be cremated and their ashes spread on the waters of the Atlantic Ocean.

During the final White Night, Jones had radioed Phil Blakey to pick him and his entourage up at the mouth of the Waini River, about thirty miles north. It is important that this message was not in code because Jones knew that his radio communications were being monitored by the Federal Communication Commission, after they had received numerous complaints from the Amateur Radio Relay League about the temple's changes of frequency and other illegal uses of the airwaves. Blakey knew this was just a diversion, so he ignored Jones's message and remained in Trinidad, while anyone who might be hunting for Jones was at the mouth of the Waini River, miles from where he really was.

Jones, several trusted nurses, and about thirty armed guards set out on foot for the thirteen-mile walk to Venezuela, on a trail they had blazed earlier. The next morning, a radio communication from a Venezuelan Air Force pilot patrolling the Guyana border, was intercepted. The pilot reported seeing forty or fifty armed people crossing into Venezuela at precisely the place and time to indicate that they had come from Jonestown. The Venezuelan government would not confirm their pilot's report and understandably so. They were furious with the United States at having deceived them into giving up their land claim against Guyana based solely on an American outpost on the border that self destructed less than a month later. Thirty-five years later, Venezuela is still angry with the United States.

Jones's entourage proceeded to an isolated airstrip, boarded a plane, and flew to Africa. Jones had never been to Africa, but had three very good sources of information on just where to go and what to do. First, there was Gordon Lindsay, who, despite Jones's claims to the contrary, spent his four months in Guyana, in Jonestown, according to surviving Jonestown residents who told the FBI that they had seen him there. Lindsay had a lifetime of covering African conflicts and knew the continent well. Then there was Phil Blakey who had a lot of experience in Africa, but mostly in Angola. Then there was Frank Terpil who had supplied the armaments for both the Shalom Project and Jonestown. Terpil knew Africa well, especially Uganda, where his close personal friend, Idi Amin, was dictator.

Jones's plane landed in Uganda and the nurses and a few guards disembarked. They made their way to a village in central Uganda that was no more than a truck stop with gas pumps and prostitutes. They set up a free health clinic that was welcomed by the locals, most of whom had never seen a doctor. Prostitutes suffering from malaria, venereal disease, and other ailments lined up at the clinic for their free examinations, during which each was infected with the HIV virus in needles that drew their blood or gave them a smallpox vaccine. The prostitutes infected the truck drivers who, in turn, spread the virus throughout Africa.

Jones's deployment techniques are why AIDS began as a homosexual disease in the US and a heterosexual disease in Africa.

Jones stayed in Uganda only long enough to refuel the plane and flew on to, of all places, Israel. This is where the ham radio operators lost his trail.

What, if anything, Jones sold to the Israelis is not known, but it is worth noting that today one-third of all Palestinian women in the disputed territories are HIV-positive. In two or three more generations, there will be no dispute in these regions, because there will be no Palestinians.

Jim Jones was forty-seven years old, free from his wife and previous identity, well-connected, and immensely wealthy. The world was his for the taking.

# F O U R T E E N

## SANCTIONED ASSASSINATIONS

*"Three can keep a secret, if two of them are dead."*

—Benjamin Franklin.

The killings were not confined to Jonestown. The CIA sanctioned at least a dozen executions of people who were close enough to Jones to at least suspect that he worked for them. Jim Jones had killed a US congressman and launched a worldwide pandemic that would kill millions. The agency had to be absolutely certain that no one remained to associate them with his crimes.

Before the experiments in Jonestown could proceed, it was essential that anyone from Jones's CIA past be eliminated. The list was short, Dan Mitrione, Jones's childhood friend, who had initially recruited him under the "buddy system" into the CIA, and Richard Welch, the US ambassador to British Guiana, who was Jones's handler for his early work in Guiana's transition from British rule to CIA rule, through their puppet Prime Minister Forbes Burnham.

Mitrione had outlived his usefulness, having taught his torture techniques to just about everyone who mattered. On August 10, 1970, Mitrione was kidnapped in Uruguay where he was teaching the police there how to interrogate and torture their citizens. A ransom note, supposedly from a group called the Tupamaros, demanded the release of 150 of their own who were in prison. The Tupamaros were a group of middle class professionals; bankers, doctors and lawyers, whose major crimes to date had been stealing incriminating government documents and forwarding them to the courts. The Tupamaros were not angels, but they were not militants either. They had kidnapped officials for ransom before, but they only wanted justice from a corrupt government. When they robbed a bank, they demanded that those citizens in line be allowed to deposit their money so the financial loss would be borne by the bank exclusively. On one occasion, they robbed a casino. In the next day's news, the casino's employees complained that they had taken their tip money as well, so the Tupamaros returned that portion to the casino. These modern day Robin Hoods were a pain in the Uruguayan government's side and Mitrione was helping them extract information from known members. The ransom note, that was probably written by the CIA, was ignored, and Mitrione's body was dumped with a bullet hole in his head. Uruguay used the murder to suspend civil rights. All suspected Tupamaros were arrested and tortured until they revealed every last member. All were killed. No one was ever accused of Mitrione's murder. The White House and the State Department sent patriotic red, white, and blue flower arrangements to his family. The Secretary of State and President Nixon's son-in-law attended Mitrione's funeral. About a week after the funeral, Mitrione's brother received a phone call from Frank Sinatra, who along with Jerry Lewis, offered to host a benefit concert in Richmond, Indiana to raise money for Mitrione's widow and nine children. Sinatra paid for everything. Over 4,000 attended. It was a gala event with food, music, dancing and gambling on 50/50 raffles. Everyone enjoyed the evening that was reminiscent of a large Italian wedding, less the bride and groom.

It was about this time that the CIA's 201 employment file on Jones was purged. It was an attempt to erase his history, but oddly, they kept the file folder with his name on it, but there was nothing left inside.

Richard Welch presented a different problem. He had a long distinguished career with the State Department. He was a valuable asset and so was allowed to live and be used until the last possible moment. On December 23, 1975, as Jones prepared to move to Guyana and start the experiments, Richard Welch, the recently appointed US ambassador to Greece, answered a knock on his front door and was fatally shot once in the head. A note, supposedly from a left-wing group called the November 17 Movement, claimed responsibility but no one was ever arrested. Welch's death required a more dignified approach. CIA Director William Colby petitioned President Ford to make an exception and allow Welch to be buried, with full military honors, in Arlington Cemetery, even though he did not die in military service. The **Washington Post** called it, "a show of pomp usually reserved for the nation's most renowned military heroes." Welch's body was carried to Arlington on the same caisson that had carried President Kennedy's body. Director Colby blamed Welch's death on leaked information about his CIA career, recently published in *Counterspy Magazine* and **The Village Voice**. It was fodder for Colby's cannon that he fired at Congress to enact the "Agent Identities Protection Act," making it a felony to expose an employee of the CIA. Coming on the heels of Welch's murder, it easily passed into law and discouraged the exposure of thousands of CIA operatives, including one named

Jim Jones. This was William Colby's last official act. The next week he was fired. They did not kill him, at least not yet.

Both of these assassinations were so similar as to indicate a common assassin. Both were killed because they were CIA, both died execution style, both murders were blamed on left leaning groups, no one was ever arrested, and both murders remain unsolved. But, what is extraordinary, is that in both cases, the CIA uncharacteristically admitted that they worked for them which they never, ever do. Their number one rule is never divulge that someone is a CIA operative.

Flash forward to the days immediately following Jonestown. San Franciscans were reeling from the ascending body count in the headlines, but none more than Mayor George Moscone and Supervisor Harvey Milk. Jones had supported Moscone and opposed Milk and because of their close encounters, both men knew that Jones was working for the CIA. Moscone tried to put on a brave face, but Milk panicked. He spent his last days as any condemned man would do, settling the business of his life. He knew the CIA was about to kill him. Milk was not paranoid- they **really were** out to get him. He had about a week to live.

Congressman Ryan's body was brought back to San Francisco for his funeral. There is no indication that Milk attended, he was probably too afraid. Despite the fact that the FBI had warned Moscone that he may be a target for assassination, he had to go to the funeral, after all, he was the mayor. As Moscone rounded the public sidewalk to enter the church, a woman grabbed his arm to escort him in. Newspaper reports claimed that the "unidentified woman scared the daylights out of him." According to her book, that "unidentified woman" was Bonnie Malmin, Jones's interpreter in his early work in Brazil and Mayor Moscone's "escort" to Peoples Temple services in San Francisco. Bonnie sat with Moscone in the church and tried to intimidate him into remaining silent about Jones. As they listened to Ryan's attorney, Joe Holsinger, give the eulogy, Malmin whispered that she would expose Moscone as an adulterer and ruin his career and family, if he said anything about Jones. Moscone would not be swayed, not even after Malmin introduced him to a woman identified only as "Sister Barbara." Sister Barbara wore a lapel pin that read "Hitler was Right" in Hebrew. Moscone was so shaken by the encounter with Malmin that he skipped the burial and went straight home and locked the door, but Bonnie's work had just begun.

Bonnie Malmin somehow managed to board the bus reserved for the congressmen who had flown from Washington DC to pay respect to their fallen colleague. On the trip to the National Cemetery in San Bruno, at the grave site, and all the way back, Malmin quizzed every congressman on the bus, trying to determine if anyone suspected more about the assassination than was reported in the press.

Back in San Francisco, Ryan's family had reserved a hotel room for a private reception. Again, Malmin managed to gain access. At the reception were thirty-eight grieving relatives and Malmin asking each if they suspected anything about Ryan's death that had not been reported. Only Ryan's daughter, Patricia, responded that she was certain her father had been killed by the CIA. She could not have come up to speed on such a complicated subject in just the few days since her father's death. Ryan had left her a detailed "In Case of My Death" letter before he set out to investigate what he knew was a CIA operation. In any event, she intended to sue the CIA. Killing her after her accusations and so soon after killing her father, would have raised too many suspicions. They had to approach her lawsuit with more finesse.

After filing her final report to the CIA, in a dramatic move, Malmin literally checked herself into a nunnery to write her memoirs. Back in Belo Horizonte, Brazil, she was first introduced as Bonnie Malmin. In the end, she was Bonnie Malmin Burnham Theilman. Her first husband was obviously named Burnham, but his identity and possible relationship to Forbes Burnham has never been revealed.

Nine days after Jonestown, Mayor George Moscone and City Supervisor Harvey Milk were assassinated; each with one gunshot to the head, execution style, which would be the hallmark of all the CIA murders that took place on US soil.

Two months later, Josep Mengele drowned in Bertioga, Brazil, while supposedly swimming in the Atlantic Ocean. Mengele's handlers had rented a beach house for him to vacation from his many problems. Years of running and hiding had taken its toll on Mengele. Even his brief periods of peace were spent at manual labor on isolated farms, where he was hidden from the outside world. He was in his late sixties, paranoid and depressed at never having received the recognition he felt he deserved. He complained constantly about his poor health and degenerative spine, that caused him severe back pain. His companions later reported that Mengele had a stroke and drowned, despite their attempts to save him. He was buried a few miles away in the town of Embu under the name of his handler, Wolfgang Gerhard. It was not until 1985 that the body was exhumed and positively identified as Mengele. No one ever questioned what an old, frail man with a bad back and no history of even being able to swim, was doing in the strong undertow of the Atlantic surf.

Immediately after Mengele's death, the US Justice Department established the Office of Special Investigations charged with identifying and expelling German Nazis from the United States. Why now? These Nazis had been in the United States for thirty-four years. What was the impetus for expelling them now? It was Jonestown. The Justice Department realized that they had been fooled, but they were not going to be fooled again.

It took a few years for the federal government to fully appreciate the damage done in Jonestown. It was only then that it understood the scope of the pandemic and they panicked. Anyone, everyone, even those just suspected of being an agent of a foreign government, were arrested and deported. Hundreds, perhaps thousands of people were escorted out of the country in 1985, in what historians have dubbed, "The Year of the Spy".

Four months after Jonestown, on March 13,1979, Jones's press secretary, Michael Prokes, was shot dead during a press conference he had called in Modesto, California, to disclose that he and Jones were working for the CIA. Several invited reporters crowded into a Motel 6 room and were each given Prokes's eleven-page manifesto that may have survived, but has never been published. He admitted to being on the CIA's payroll and even identified his handler as a "Mr. Jackson". When asked if Jones worked for the CIA as well, Prokes knew it would be a long, complicated explanation, so he first excused himself, walked into the bathroom, and locked the door. A gunshot rang out. By the time the reporters broke down the door, they found Prokes dead on the floor from a single gunshot wound to the head. Police recorded his death as the suicide of a remorseful man, caught up in a terrible situation.

At first it would appear to be an open and shut case, but it was really a locked room, Sherlock Holmes mystery. The CIA often refers to assassinations as "wet work" because of the blood. In this case, they utilized a "wet wall." In inexpensive multi-residential structures, like a Motel 6, plumbing is shared by adjoining occupancies through a wet wall that contains the water supply lines, the vent and drain for the bathrooms that are mirror images of each other. The toilets are back to back, the vanities are back to back, and the medicine cabinets are back to back. Remove the medicine cabinet from the room next door and you are looking at the plastic backside of the adjoining room's medicine cabinet. Prokes had to invite the media days earlier so there was ample time for the CIA to rent the room next door, remove the medicine cabinet, and hinge Prokes's cabinet to swing open. At a predetermined signal, the assassin opened the cabinet, shot Prokes in the head, threw the gun into the room, secured both cabinets, and was conceivably driving out of the parking lot before the reporters were able to break down the door. No one checked for Prokes's fingerprints on the gun or conducted nitrate tests on his hands. After all, it was a locked room, an open and shut case.

Elmer and Deanna Mertle were two Caucasians who were heavily into the Civil Rights Movement. Elmer had even walked by Martin Luther King's side on his famous march from Selma to Montgomery, Alabama. They had relocated to California and were attracted to Jones's public persona as the charismatic leader of a multi-racial, socialistic utopian culture. They wanted to join the Peoples Temple, but Jones never wanted them, though they did have certain skills he could use, at least temporarily. Deanna was a professional-grade writer and Jones put her to work writing temple literature. Elmer became the temple's photographer. The Mertles had invited themselves and, eventually, Jones wanted them out, so he devised a plan to force them to leave voluntarily. Reportedly, Jones spanked their daughter, Daphene, over seventy times with a wooden paddle. Aside from the sadistic pleasure that Jones enjoyed repeatedly spanking a sixteen- year-old girl, the incident served to finally convince the Mertles, who were apparently somewhat naive and thick-headed, to leave the Peoples Temple. They moved to the East Bay and started an organization to help deprogram former cult members. Their group evolved into the "Concerned Relatives." They hired Joe Mazor, a private investigator, to gather as much dirt on Jim Jones as he could. Deborah Layton, Tim Carter, and Tim Stoen, who were all still working for Jones, joined the Concerned Relatives to use the group to convince Congressman Ryan to investigate Jonestown. Elmer and Deanna had since legally changed their names to Al and Jeannie Mills, in order to avoid any repercussions from having signed the blank piece of paper that was Jones's test of loyalty.

The CIA needed to know what the Mertles or now the "Mills" knew, so they looked to their closest asset for an answer. Tim Stoen suggested that Jeannie write a book. Stoen took care of everything. He found Jeannie an agent, a publisher, and a rather generous $30,000 advance on royalties. She used the money to buy a Mercedes Benz. Jeannie Mills told everything she knew about Jones in her book, entitled *Six Years With God,* but she had no control over its publication. Stoen had arranged for the copyright to be held by an untraceable group called MBR investments, who edited Jeannie's text that was published by A&W Publishing. There was only one press run. MBR investments and A&W Publishing immediately declared bankruptcy. Thirty days after publication, an unknown assassin entered the Mills home and shot Al, Jeannie, and their daughter, once in the head, execution style. All of the murders in the US were professional hits; one small caliber bullet to the head, no misses, no struggle, nothing taken, no evidence left, no one charged; all unsolved.

Dr. Walter Rodney was an internationally recognized, award-winning, Caribbean historian and scholar who returned to his native Guyana to investigate the Guyana government's involvement in Jonestown. On June 13, 1980, an officer with the Guyanese Defense Force offered Rodney inside information about Jim Jones. He gave him a walkie-talkie and told him to stand by for further instructions. The phone rang, he put it to his ear, and it exploded, blowing his head off.

Paula Adams was a very attractive young Caucasian aide to Jones, who he appointed as the temple's ambassador to the Guyana government. She developed a close personal relationship with Guyana's ambassador to the US, Lawrence Mann, and after Jonestown, the two moved to Bethesda, Maryland, where they parented a daughter. In 1983, an unknown assassin entered their Maryland home and shot Paula Adams, Lawrence Mann, and their daughter once in the head. Paula and Lawrence knew too much, their innocent daughter was collateral damage, or perhaps not. Offspring of their targets, like Patricia Ryan, were already giving them problems.

In late 1985, Prime Minister Forbes Burnham died under suspicious circumstances after simple throat surgery. The operation was a success and Burnham appeared to be on the mend, but several days later, he succumbed to something that has only been described as "complications."

The Concerned Relatives were gone, but the private detective they had hired was so intrigued by the story that he continued to investigate Jim Jones on his own. In 1986, Joe Mazor was killed in California— shot once in the head by an unknown assassin.

The last in this series of sanctioned assassinations may well have been the death of William Colby where this story began.

These were not revenge killings. None of these people ever did anything to hurt Jones or the CIA. Actually, many of them helped him. Even Al and Jeannie Mills's creation of the Concerned Relatives group helped Jones entice Ryan to his death, which was exactly what he wanted. These victims were murdered, not for what they **did** to Jones, but for what they **knew** about Jones. They **knew** he was CIA. The Company was just covering its tracks.

# F I F T E E N

## DAMAGE CONTROL

*"I can turn a triangle into a square if I just repeat it enough."*

—Dr. Joseph Goebbels, Nazi Germany's
Reich Minister of Propaganda.

Never before had the CIA been embroiled in so much controversy as they were over Jonestown. Not even after their failed Bay of Pigs invasion of Cuba or accusations that they had assassinated President Kennedy and Martin Luther King, were they under as much intense scrutiny and pressure. The stated story of Jonestown just did not make any sense. There had to be something more. The people of Guyana wanted answers. Foreign governments, that had long since accepted that Guyana was controlled by the CIA, wanted to know how 900 Americans and a US congressman were killed on the CIA's watch. Everyone from the President of the United States, to Congress, to the FBI, to the American public were hammering the CIA for answers. The Agency was killing all the witnesses and destroying as much evidence as possible, but they still had to spin a massive disinformation campaign just to survive the assault. Jones had begun the media blitz a month earlier in October, 1978, when he instructed his attorney, Mark Lane, to hold a press conference to announce that his client intended to sue just about every agency of the US federal government for harassment. Named in the proposed lawsuit that Jones said would be filed in ninety days, was the CIA, The State Department, the FBI, the IRS, the Treasury Department, the Federal Communications Commission, and the US Postal Service. This was all just Jones's attempt to distance himself from his government sponsors, though it is true that he was being pressured by the FCC and the USPS after they had received numerous complaints about his illegal use of the airwaves and his tampering with the mail. Jones confiscated or censored all letters either into or out of Jonestown. The proposed lawsuit was just an idle threat. Jones knew that ninety days later, Jonestown would not even exist. The most common form of brainwashing is propaganda, and the propaganda was flowing like a fountain from both Jones and the CIA.

The CIA's first order of business was to destroy all evidence at the scene of the crime. A few days after the murder/suicides, Prime Minister Forbes Burnham addressed the Guyana National Parliament to defend his association with Jones, but his speech was drowned out by cries of, "Shame! Cover up! Shame! Cover up!." Obviously, Burnham had lost the confidence of his government, but he was prepared for the political backlash, having postponed scheduled elections in 1978 citing the need for a new constitution. Guyana's chief justice was given the ultimate authority to conduct an investigation into the government's involvement with Jonestown. He subpoenaed any and all records that were then stored in a Georgetown warehouse. Once the warehouse was stuffed with thousands of pounds of contracts, communications, and reports from Jonestown, it was burned to the ground. Eyewitnesses reported that the arsonists wore Guyanese Defense Forces uniforms. Burnham also ordered that Jonestown be totally destroyed by fire, nothing was to be salvaged, nothing saved. He was particularly interested in destroying the mattresses. He did not want the locals to reuse them. He knew enough about the experiment to suspect that the mattresses might be contaminated. All the evidence in Guyana had been destroyed, but there were still problems. After a few days to determine whether they had legal jurisdiction, the FBI assembled a team that they intended to send to Guyana. Even though this happened overseas, the FBI was within its legal rights to investigate the deaths of 900 Americans and a US congressman. The CIA would not tolerate FBI interference and so instructed their puppet prime minister to bar all FBI personnel from entering Guyana. In Guyana, there would be no US government investigation into Jonestown or the death of a congressman.

The CIA got a windfall break shortly after Ryan's murder when the second phase of the Hughes-Ryan Amendment came up for vote in Congress. It was soundly defeated. Apparently, very few on Capital Hill were willing to champion Ryan's cause, lest they suffer a similar fate.

Ryan's daughter presented a serious problem. Patricia Ryan had filed a $68 million dollar lawsuit against the CIA, Director Stansfield Turner, Mike Prokes, Phil Blakey, and Dick Dwyer, claiming that they were all a part of a "mass mind-control CIA experiment" that killed her father. The CIA did not care about the money. They cared about the publicity of a court proceeding that could find them responsible for assassinating a congressman. By then, Mike Prokes was dead, Phil Blakey could not be extradited from Angola, and Turner was so insulated that he was untouchable and, so that left only Dick Dwyer. After graduating from Princeton, Dwyer went to work for the State

Department's Bureau of Intelligence and Research, followed by postings in Damascus, Cairo, and Sofia. He was the CIA station chief in Bangkok during the Vietnam War and now in Guyana. Prime Minister Forbes Burnham was just a figurehead. The real head of government in Guyana was the CIA and the CIA was Dick Dwyer. Dwyer's career with the CIA and his relationship with Jones were indefensible. As a last ditch effort, the State Department awarded Dwyer a medal for his "heroic actions" at the airstrip. Dwyer's actions at the airstrip could hardly be considered "heroic." He first made certain that the victims were disarmed and could not defend themselves. Only one gunman approached to do the killing. Dwyer had a shotgun, but instead of killing the lone assassin, he handed his weapon to him, that he used to kill Ryan and the others. Dwyer ignored the pleas of the wounded, failed to defend Ryan, and then ordered the only functioning plane back to Georgetown, with just the pilots and Monica Bagby on board and several empty seats that could have carried the seriously wounded out of harm's way and back to Georgetown for much needed medical treatment. Dwyer then confiscated and withheld evidence from the dead at the airstrip; evidence in the murder of a US congressman that would never see the light of day. Dwyer should have been arrested, not given a medal, but the CIA was drowning and desperately grasping at straws.

Patricia Ryan's wrongful death lawsuit could not be allowed to proceed. At pretrial disclosure hearings, the CIA stalled when asked for information. They stalled and stalled and stalled and then had the audacity to ask the judge to dismiss the suite on the grounds that Patricia Ryan had not prosecuted in a timely fashion. Their tactic worked and the case was dismissed, but that was not enough for the CIA spin doctors, they needed to be certain that Ryan's children would not raise any more objections, so they set out on a massive smear campaign designed to discredit them. News stories circulated that Patricia Ryan and her sister had joined a cult in Oregon, run by an East Indian guru. In a separate attack, news stories claimed that Ryan's daughter worked for the CIA, but resigned, to accept a position as assistant to Congresswoman Jackie Speier, who had run for and won Ryan's vacated seat in the House of Representatives.

The State Department appointed US Attorney William Hunter to look into Jonestown and prosecute Larry Layton. From the beginning, they were trying to whitewash the proceedings. When it was revealed that Hunter had worked with Tim Stoen to suppress the investigation of the 1975 election fraud in San Francisco when both of them were assistant district attorneys,

Hunter stepped down to avoid the inevitable scandal, and appointed his assistant, Robert Dordero as lead prosecutor in Layton's trial.

News article after news article referred to the "drug crazed California cult leader." The CIA pounded this message into the common American experience. People tended to dismiss the event as insanity and not the cold-hearted, calculated medical experiment that it really was. The words, "mass suicide" were repeated so many times that thirty-five years later, Americans still believe it, despite the fact that the only forensic examination of the bodies, done by Guyana's Chief Coroner concluded that most of the victims had been murdered. Murder indicates that someone was responsible and that was the last thing the CIA wanted because it leads to the question, "Who?" By calling it a mass suicide, there was no one left to blame. Even small details like the cyanide-laced drink were changed. It was not Kool-Aid, it was Flavor-Aid, but Flavor-Aid was not as familiar to the American public as Kool-Aid, so they changed it so all of the references and jokes for the last thirty-five years have been technically incorrect.

Something very extraordinary happened next. The CIA was called to task. This could only have come from the president. Knowledge of the Jonestown Project was so compartmentalized that only a small cell within the Agency knew, but now, as their defenses crumbled, it became increasingly apparent that the entire agency was about to be blamed. The CIA plea bargained. They could never admit to killing a congressman, but they did agree to make certain concessions. On December 4, 1980, the **New York Times** published two articles on the same page; "House Committee Clears C.I.A. of Role in People's Temple" and "C.I.A. Linked to Mind-Control Drug Experiments." By admitting to their involvement in **MK ULTRA** while denying their involvement in Jonestown, the CIA gave the impression that these were two different subjects when they were, in fact, the same story. Meanwhile, researchers were misdirected towards **MK ULTRA** and away from Jonestown.

Whether they created the AIDS epidemic or not, the CIA realized that they needed to defend themselves for sponsoring a project that did create it. They found it relatively easy to manipulate the news media if they just did their work for them. Produce a well-written, somewhat believable article, and newspapers will publish it, without too many questions.

To defend themselves against allegations that they had created AIDS, the CIA took a three pronged approach:

—Establish that the HIV virus was the natural evolution of a green monkey virus, even though there is no scientific basis for this and there are no monkeys or apes in the wild with AIDS, but this helped to take the heat off claims that the virus was manmade. If the HIV virus was natural, it would have infected mankind universally, but it did not. Initially, it targeted only young, otherwise healthy, gay men in Manhattan. The virus is too perfect and too targeted to have randomly evolved in nature. This implies an intelligence not possessed by viruses.

—"AIDS was God's revenge against sinful homosexuals." This modern day Sodom and Gomorrah rationale may sound absurd to most people, but it was taken very seriously by about a third of Americans. Once the name of God is evoked, there is no reason for some people to look any further. This tactic was effective, but it did not explain the heterosexual transmission of the disease in Africa.

—AIDS predated 1978. The CIA placed hundreds of articles claiming there was evidence of AIDS prior to 1978. Typical of these was their claim that an African native exhibited AIDS-like symptoms after being bitten by a monkey back in the 1950s. There was a period of time when every newspaper article about AIDS attempted to date the origin of the virus prior to 1978. It was a blitz campaign, but then it just stopped abruptly because it was supported by lies that could not stand the test of time. The Center for Disease Control accurately established that the technology to create the virus was perfected in 1977 and AIDS first appeared in late 1978.

With all the witnesses dead and the evidence destroyed and enough "wild goose chases" established, the CIA fell silent. They had done a terrible disservice to those who were searching for the origin of the virus. Most researchers refused to challenge the scientific status quo, and set out in the wrong direction, while the pandemic spread like wildfire, claiming millions of lives.

# S I X T E E N

## DRUGS AND MONEY

*"Follow the Money."*

**—Informant "Deep Throat's" advice to reporters Woodward and Bernstein who were investigating the Watergate scandal.**

Jim Jones was born into poverty, but when he disappeared at age 47, he was worth somewhere between $52 million and $2 billion dollars. Estimates vary widely because he was extremely skilled at hiding his assets behind dummy front companies, foreign real estate investments, anonymous numbered bank accounts, and large foreign safety deposit boxes. His total worth will never be known, but it suffices to say that it was significant.

The federal government continued to provide financial support to Jones even after he moved his people to Guyana. Jones had carefully selected only 1,200 out of his 5,000 followers to immigrate to Guyana based upon, among other things, their Social Security benefits. Each received a monthly pension or disability check of about one thousand dollars, times an average of 1,000 residents deposited $1 million into Jones's coffers every month. The residents never saw the money. All their basic needs of food, clothing, shelter and energy were provided, besides, in the remote jungle, there was nowhere for them to spend money. Since the experiment was active for over twenty-five months, Jones took the entire $25 million in 1978 money, that today is worth more than the gross national product of most third world countries.

In January, 1979, the Justice Department initiated a $4.2 million dollar lawsuit against the Peoples Temple to recover the cost of returning the bodies to the US. The lawsuit was not only about the money, it was intended to distance the federal government from their responsibilities. Robert Fabian was appointed receiver or quasi-executor of the temple's estate. It took him a year to uncover a few foreign accounts that he reported were worth $10 million dollars. Since this amount was sufficient to settle the Justice Department's lawsuit, he stopped looking after only having scratched the surface.

Jones hid his money in trusts that would invest in foreign companies that would deposit the money into other foreign companies that would deposit money into yet other foreign banks. Uncovering his assets presented an almost impossible task of petitioning the court systems of several different countries before arriving at the one whose banks held the money. In the years that followed, independent researchers and media reporters have uncovered at least eighteen additional secret accounts in Switzerland, Panama, the Bahamas, Grenada, Venezuela, the Virgin Islands, Trinidad, and France that totaled more than $30 million dollars. There are other reports of more accounts in Panama and a $17 million dollar real estate investment. Fabian preferred to glean temple assets that were more readily accessible. He sold the temple's headquarters in San Francisco for $300,000 and placed liens on other temple real estate valued at $2.5 million. He tried to seize the *Albatross* that was docked in Trinidad at the time, but the Justice Department refused his suggestion after Dr. Lawrence Layton interceded on behalf of his soon to be ex-son-in-law, Phil Blakey, who was living on the ship. Only then did Blakey way anchor and sail to Africa to continue his work in Angola and avoid extradition back to the US and Patricia Ryan's lawsuit that awaited him. According to Mark Lane's testimony to the FBI, the ship carried an extremely large amount of cash.

Early on, back in California, attorney Tim Stoen had warned Jones that his money was piling up so fast that it could draw unwanted attention and raise questions as to how he acquired it. Later on, this advice was still pertinent, but the dollar amounts were much greater. Jones instructed his top aides, Terri Buford, Deborah Layton, and Maria Katsaris to research the banking laws of several foreign countries. The three traveled to Panama, Venezuela, London, Paris, Switzerland, France, Romania, and the Cayman Islands to set up dummy companies, open bank accounts and rent safety deposit boxes. Since the object was to hide the money, only a few accounts were in the name of the Peoples Temple. Most were in the names of the three woman or phony investment companies that they had set up to manage Jones's estate. Corporations, like Bridget, S.A., Angelique, and Asociacion Religiosa Pro San Pedro, S.A., that were managed by Jones from afar, deposited large sums of cash into accounts that were virtually untraceable. The largest sums were deposited into numbered Swiss accounts or Swiss safety deposit boxes, where not even the banks knew the contents. The Swiss government admitted that a few accounts were transferred to the United States after Jonestown's demise, but they would not say to whom, citing the 1973 US-Swiss Legal Assistance Treaty.

One of the Swiss accounts was in the name of Annie McGowan, a Jonestown resident, who along with Maria Katsaris, died on the final day. That left only Terri Buford and Deborah Layton knowing where the money was hidden. Buford moved in with attorney Mark Lane and allegedly, the two traveled to Switzerland to empty accounts that were either numbered or in Buford's name. This could be seen as repayment for the Shalom Project that was headed by Buford's father and managed by Jones. After Jonestown's demise, Deborah Layton divorced Phil Blakey and married temple aide Mike Cartmell and settled into her new job as a money manager in San Francisco's financial district. Her position flew in the face of her rather mediocre high school education and begged the questions, "Whose money was she managing? Was it hers? It would have been appropriate for Jones to repay the seed money provided by Deborah's grandfather, Nazi banker Hugo Philip.

Jones had deposited $2 million dollars in the National Cooperative Bank of Guyana as collateral for the land lease. On the day after the massacre, Guyana's first lady, Viola Burnham, reportedly took $1 million dollars cash from Jones's cabin. Mark Lane later reported to the FBI that there was at least $3 million dollars in cash in Jones's cabin. Fabian conceded that all this money belonged to Guyana to compensate them for the project.

The upper estimate of Jones's wealth at $2 billion would seem to be unobtainable until one considers another aspect of his secret life; trafficking illegal drugs.

Jones was pleased to be remembered as a paranoid drug addict because it helped to explain the events of the final White Night, but all references to his alleged drug habit came from Jones himself and he is not to be believed. If anything, Jones had a heightened awareness of the dangers of drugs. He controlled the minds of a thousand people and could not have accomplished that without being in total control of his own. He was sober, clear-headed, and determined.

With Jones's South American connections, immunity from prosecution, ability to travel undetected under a second passport, and desire to amass as much wealth as possible without regard for human suffering, illegal drugs would have been attractive to him. According to the Brazilian newspaper, **Manchete**, South American law enforcement agencies were investigating allegations that Jones was trafficking drugs between Bolivia, Brazil and Guyana in the early 1960s as was his employer, INVESCO. INVESCO was suspected of dealing in heroin, but, if Bolivia was the source, cocaine was the drug. Bolivia's constitution guarantees the right of its citizens to legally grow coca plants, the leaves of which they chew for a mild stimulant, but those leaves can also be processed into cocaine. It would have been easy and legal for Jones to purchase large quantities of coca leaves in Bolivia and transport it over the rather porous border with Brazil to a town like Mato Grosso where it could be processed into cocaine. A decade later, in 1972, a CIA report placed Josep Mengele in Mato Grosso where they said he was involved in drug trafficking. Back in Germany, Mengele's family had stopped supporting the black sheep of their family. Mengele was broke and Jones may have come to his aid by giving him his old Mato Grosso processing plant.

A US soldier with the "Graves Registration Detachment" assigned to clean up the bodies in Jonestown, reported to the FBI that he had the opportunity to review temple records in Jonestown before they were confiscated by Guyanese authorities and he found evidence of drug trafficking. His report was confirmed by the FBI's New York office, and the US Coast Guard in Miami, Florida.

Jones was not smuggling drugs in a suitcase and selling them on a street corner. This was large scale brokering. He probably never saw the product, he only had to move money and contacts. The drug enforcement authorities in South America ended their trail in Guyana because that is where their jurisdiction ended, but that was not the final destination. Guyana is a poor country, not a consumer country. The ultimate destination was the United States. It was relatively easy for Jones to smuggle drugs into the US in the early 1960s because law enforcement was primitive by today's standard, but he needed one single customer that was as large as his shipments. Organized crime was the only answer. With one investment, Jones could turn a million dollars into a billion dollars.

There may have been another reason why Jones moved to Mendocino County in California. Mendocino has a world-wide reputation for producing the highest quality wines and marijuana. Actually, Mendocino County produces more marijuana than any other region of the country. Jones, who controlled the entire county, could not have ignored what was California's largest agricultural cash crop growing right outside his door. He had lost his South American suppliers, but not his US customers, who he could now supply with marijuana. He would have kept a safe distance from the operation, having his minions purchase the harvests of local farmers and ship it back east, at a tremendous profit.

The purpose of the Shalom Project was to support the UNITA rebels in Angola that needed black, Portuguese-speaking mercenaries, arms, and supplies. The CIA could provide these things, but it had no assurance that the rebels would accept them. They needed more. UNITA rebels had a reputation for smoking marijuana, so along with the mercenaries, guns, supplies, and food, the agency sent marijuana that Phil Blakey grew at the Guyana encampment. Excess production was shipped to the US to further add to Jones's coffers.

After four days in the jungle heat, the bodies in Jonestown had swelled from expanding internal gases. The Guyanese Defense Forces bayoneted the corpses from throat to genitals to release the gas. Local Guyanese reported that two kilos of heroin were then stuffed into each of the body cavities before they were placed into the airtight aluminum coffins. Supposedly, the coffins were not opened during the trip to Dover Air Force Base and then onto California but a billion dollars could have changed that.

Only the President of the United States knows the amount of the CIA's annual secret "black budget," but not even the president knows how that money is spent. He is presented with a nondescript, line item request. He can ask questions about this line or that, but the scope of the operation is so large that no single human being could ever comprehend it all and, even if he could, he has no assurance that the funds would be spent on that project or some other. Furthermore, there are no checks to prevent the CIA from using that money to make more money. This has lead to speculation that the CIA is involved in illegal activities like trafficking drugs in order to finance projects that cannot be traced, even by the president. There may be some truth to these allegations but there is definite proof that the CIA turns a blind eye to trafficking drugs by their operatives. In a 1975 Senate Committee meeting, it was confirmed that the CIA knowingly allowed one of their operatives to smuggle twenty-five kilos of heroin into the United States unabated. It is a symbiotic relationship, an honor among thieves. The CIA knows the crimes of its operatives and its operatives know the crimes of the CIA. It is all 'wink-wink, hush-hush,' at least until it makes front page news.

# SEVENTEEN

## THE KIDNAPPING OF PATTY HEARST

*"I cry easily. I wept every time I read about Patty Hearst. I thought, there but for the grace of God go I and then it all happened to me."*

**—Dr. Lawrence Layton in a statement to the San Francisco Chronicle after Jonestown's demise.**

In one well calculated defense, Dr. Layton painted himself as a god-fearing, compassionate humanitarian when, in fact, he was a cold-hearted germ warfare scientist who spent most of his career devising new ways to kill vast numbers of people, but he was also sending a message to the CIA to leave him and his family alone or he would expose that they had kidnapped and brainwashed millionaire heiress Patty Hearst.

Congressman Leo Ryan first crossed paths with the CIA's **MK ULTRA** project and Jim Jones at the intersection of Patty Hearst's kidnapping.

It all started when Ryan accused the CIA of conducting illegal operations in his home district. Innocent citizens were being harmed and Ryan was mad as hell. Surprisingly, the CIA admitted to running operatives in Ryan's San Mateo County and adjacent Santa Clara County, but convinced him it was necessary for national security. It was not until years later, that President Ronald Reagan amended the CIA's charter to allow them to operate in country, but at the time, the entire concept of the CIA operating on US soil was illegal, but apparently justified. The region that came to be known as Silicon Valley was a vast treasure house of classified military, industrial and technological secrets, that both enemy and friendly countries coveted. There were more foreign spies in Silicone Valley than there were in Washington, D.C., Moscow and Beijing combined. Add to that mix an equal number of US counter intelligence operatives and the result was a complicated, tangled mess of intrigue, coercion, bribery, blackmail, kidnapping and murder.

Satisfied that the CIA's counter intelligence operations in his home district were necessary, Ryan shifted his attention to allegations the CIA was using mind control techniques learned from their **MK ULTRA** experiments to establish cults in California. He first concentrated on Sun Myung Moon's Unification Church, but the CIA put an immediate and unexplained stop to his investigation. Ryan then looked to the Symbionese Liberation Army.

There was a very strong prison reform movement in California at the time that was worthy of Ryan's attention. He even went so far as to submit to a full body search and be incarcerated, under an assumed named, in Folsom Prison for ten days to study the conditions. The foremost activist for reform within the prison system was Donald DeFreeze, a small time crook sentenced to Vacaville State Psychiatric Prison for armed robbery. Vacaville State Psychiatric Prison was the site of a CIA **MK SEARCH Subproject 3 (a division of MK ULTRA)** experiment in behavior modification conducted by Dr. James Hamilton as revealed in a letter from CIA Deputy Director Frank Carlucci to Congressman Ryan, dated October 18, 1978, exactly one month before Ryan's assassination. In 1977 and 78, Ryan had demanded specific information about the CIA's mind control experiments at Vacaville State Prison. One of their patients or "test persons" was Donald DeFreeze. Dr. Colston Westbrook, a CIA psychological warfare expert created in DeFreeze an alternative personality that could be triggered by calling him his "other name," Cinque.

DeFreeze had a small following both in and out of prison when, without explanation, he was transferred to Soledad State Prison where, in March of 1973, he escaped with "help from the outside." In August, 1973, his co-conspirator, Thero Wheeler, escaped from Vacaville Prison to complete the initial Symbionese Liberation Army or SLA that was comprised of Donald DeFreeze (Cinque), Thero Wheeler (Bayo), Willie Wolf (Cujo), Russell Little (Osceola), Joseph Remiro (Bo), Angela Atwood (General Gelina), Bill Harris (General Teko), Emily Harris (Yolanda), Patricia Soltysok (Zoya), Camilla Hall (Gabi) and Nancy Ling Perry (Fahizah).Some were **MK ULTRA** programmed assassins and together they were extremely dangerous. Oddly, the SLA was all Caucasian, except for its leader, Cinque, who was Black. Other members and sympathizers would be added later. As the legion goes, the SLA advertised their services to left wing organizations in California as a militia to advance revolutionary causes, but the truth is, since both the SLA and Jim Jones shared a common denominator in the **MK ULTRA** project a private introduction was more likely. In any event, the Symbionese Liberation Army went to work for Jim Jones.

In August of 1973, the same month that Thero Wheeler completed the SLA, Tim Stoen called a meeting in a cow pasture at the temple's Redwood

Valley ranch. The temple often conducted sensitive meetings outdoors, fearing that their buildings might have been bugged with electronic listening devices. Stoen told Patty Cartmell, Terri Buford, Sandy Bradshaw and others who would later recall the meeting, that Jones would not attend, but would be informed of the minutes of the meeting in order to maintain his deniability. There were two items on the agenda—Marcus Foster and Patty Hearst.

Tim Stoen's work in the Alameda County Juvenile Justice system, allowed him to target poor, welfare supported youths from the ghettos of Oakland who were in trouble with the law and offer them a "second chance" at a new life in the Peoples Temple in Redwood Valley. There was no shortage of black candidates from the drug and crime infested poor neighborhoods of Oakland and many accepted Stoen's offer as an attractive alternative to incarceration. The one person in a position to see the extent of this mass exodus from Oakland was Oakland City School Superintendent, Dr. Marcus Foster, and he was raising objections and asking too many questions about Stoen and Jones. He knew he was witnessing something sinister, but he did not know exactly what it was. Was it child abuse? Human trafficking? Pornography? Cult sacrifice? When in doubt, the imagination tends to go to the extreme. Foster was complaining to the authorities, contacting the press and generally calling attention to Stoen and Jones who could not survive the scrutiny. Patty Cartmell's Department of Diversions broke into Foster's home searching for information. They even went so far as to tunnel under his house to listen to his private conversations from the crawl space underneath.

Patty Hearst was not a problem, but her father was. Patty was just a weapon Jones could use to manipulate Randolph Hearst, whose newspaper, the **San Francisco Examiner** had published a series of damning articles about him and his Peoples Temple, written by their religious columnist, Episcopalian priest, Lester Kinsolving. Only four of the planned eight columns had been published, when the **Examiner** canceled the series after Jones and several hundred of his followers picketed the newspaper's offices. Jones tried to discredit Kinsolving by claiming that he was an unregistered agent of a South African country and he may well have been because, at that time, the Shalom Project was sending mercenaries from Jonestown to South Africa and retaliation could only be expected. Months later, the **Examiner** was threatening to publish another exposé and a control freak like Jones could not allow that to happen. He needed a diversion.

On November 6, 1973, Marcus Foster was shot dead, execution style, as he left a late night meeting of the Oakland School Board. The SLA claimed responsibility in a communiqué that stated they had killed Foster because he was an agent of the CIA and had plans to violate the civil rights of the Oakland students by requiring them to carry identification cards. Foster did propose such an identification card, but he was only trying to keep non-student drug dealers off school property and, besides, he had long-since withdrawn his proposal, but that was the stated reason the SLA gave for killing Foster. Perhaps it is only human nature, but this is where Jones's plan went wrong. In this world, it is not which side of the fence you are on as much as which fence you stand next to. A priest or minister is more likely to be immoral than the average person because 'morality' is their fence. The legal fence of a policeman is shared with the criminal. A New York Yankee baseball player has more in common with his arch enemy in the Boston Red Sox than he does with the general public. Jones had the SLA call Foster CIA and later called Ryan "The CIA congressman", but flipping the situation exactly 180 degrees only brings attention to the fence that both were straddling. Now it only becomes a question of who was on which side. At first, the authorities did not think the SLA even existed until a second communiqué described how Foster had been killed with a cyanide-tipped bullet, a fact the police had deliberately withheld from the public.

In January, 1974, Russell Little and Joseph Ramiro were stopped by police on a routine traffic violation and immediately arrested for murder when the officers found SLA literature in their van. That evening, their Concord, California hideout was burned to the ground by a fire of undetermined origin. With nowhere else to go, the remaining SLA hid out in the Redwood Valley home of temple guard Chris Lewis for two or three weeks.

On February 4, 1974, the SLA kidnapped Patty Hearst from her Berkeley apartment. They used Jones's Department of Diversion techniques. A woman knocked on Patty's door and asked to use the phone because her car had broken down. With the door opened, two armed men entered and subdued Patty. They waited several days before sending a communiqué in order to build suspense. Two days later, Jim Jones and aides Tim Stoen, Karen Layton, Michael Prokes and Annie Moore offered themselves as hostages in exchange for Patty Hearst in a published article in the **Press Democrat**. It was all good theater. They were in no danger, they controlled the SLA. Jones then sent a $2,000 check to the Hearst family as seed money for an anticipated ransom that never materialized. The Hearsts returned his check, but not before Jones received press coverage of his generosity.

This is when it got ugly. The San Francisco Police Department's Intelligence and Anti-terrorist Division and the FBI opened investigations into whether Jim Jones had masterminded Patty's kidnapping. This had all begun with the murder of Marcus Foster, so they asked themselves the obvious question, did Foster have any enemies, and Jim Jones was the only answer. They interviewed Jones and several of his followers. One temple member, identified only as a black woman in her mid-fifties, recognized a photo of Donald DeFreeze as someone she had seen at temple services in Redwood Valley. Jones felt sufficiently threatened by the investigation that he ordered Stoen to write a letter to the San Francisco Police Department that read, in part, "As an Assistant District Attorney, I can attest the Rev. Jones consistently... attacks scathingly...the S.L.A." Stoen went onto to say that the temple had totally disassociated itself from Chris Lewis who they suspected of harboring the SLA. Stoen told the police that Lewis had left the temple and the San Francisco Bay Area, but neglected to say that Jones had just sent him to Guyana. Privately, Jones's internal publications to his followers parroted the SLA's literature almost word for word. The SLA was not copying Jones, Jones was not copying the SLA. Both publications were written by the same hand.

Jones's first attempt to extort money from the Hearst family failed when they did not follow his lead to establish a ransom fund. Jones anticipated they would have offered a few million dollars for Patty's release that would, in turn, come back to him. When that did not materialize, the SLA demanded the Hearsts give a $70 box of food to every Californian on welfare, social security, food stamps, Medicare, parole or probation. The Hearsts refused this outrageous proposal because it accurately represented the family's 230 million dollar net worth. A compromise was struck, in which the Hearsts agreed to distribute 2 million dollars in free food to San Francisco's poor in exchange for Patty's release, after which there would be an additional 4 million dollar food giveaway.

Randolph Hearst enlisted two unlikely characters to administer the food giveaway: Washington State's Secretary, Ludlow Kramer, and Peggy Maze, director of "Neighbors in Need", a Seattle-based group formed to help subsidize unemployed aerospace workers who had lost their jobs in a massive layoff at Boeing. They formed a steering committee to oversee the distribution that included the Reverend Cecil Williams, the black pastor of San Francisco's Glide Memorial Church (who was receiving the SLA's communiqués) and American Indian Movement spokesman, Dennis Banks. At the insistence of the SLA, the committee was chaired by the Western Addition Project Area

Committee. Despite the fact that Jim Jones was the foremost advocate for the poor in San Francisco, his name was noticeably missing from the committee, but he was there, hiding in the shadows, pulling all the strings.

Jones had a close relationship with everyone on the committee. He was friends with the Reverend Cecil Williams who shared a common profession and neighborhood with Jones. Dennis Banks owed a huge dept to Jones who, just a year earlier had paid the $18,000 bail to get Bank's wife out of jail after she had been arrested by federal authorities for her part in the Wounded Knee Indian uprising. Then there was the case of the Western Addition Project Area Committee or WAPAC. It had been chaired by temple member Rory Hithe, but in an open meeting in full view of a room full of people, most of whom were temple members, temple strong arm man Chris Lewis shot and killed Hithe during a heated argument about neighborhood politics. Jones paid Lewis's legal fees and he was acquitted on grounds of self defense. Ever since that incident, Jones had total control over the WAPAC.

The plan was to distribute the food out of the back of tractor trailer trucks at unannounced, random locations in poor San Francisco neighborhoods over several weeks, but Jones knew exactly when and where, so he bussed several hundred of his followers to the locations just prior to the truck pulling up. The recipients were not required to provide identification and the accounting was strictly confined to the value of the food doled out. In one case, Jones had his aides hijack a truck on route to the giveaway and took the entire shipment. Since it was not handed out, it was not counted towards the $2 million and Jones gleaned an extra truckload. Almost all of the free food went to temple members who were instructed to bring it to the Peoples Temple Geary Street headquarters, presumably for their future consumption. Jones took all of his followers government support checks, but he still needed to feed them. There is another, more sinister possibility that is more suited to Jones's personality. He could have struck a deal with the Hearst family to save them a million dollars by recycling the food his followers received back onto trucks for the next week's free hand out, again and again, therefore making $200,000 worth of food look like $2 million. The Hearsts would save a million dollars, pay Jones $800,000 for his services plus allow him to keep the last round of $200,000 in food. This would have been the quintessential Jones, fooling everyone and playing Jesus Christ and the story of the loaves and fishes. Throughout this story, Ronald Reagan always provided comic relief and the kidnapping of Patty Hearst was no exception. At first, Reagan warned San Francisco's poor not to accept the free food, least they support the terrorist's demands, but when that failed, in a speech to congressional aides in Washington, D.C., he said he wished the recipients would, "suffer an epidemic of botulism."

As soon as this first food giveaway was over, Patty announced in a taped message to the press that she had voluntarily joined the SLA to fight the "corporate ruling class." Almost immediately, the group robbed a branch of the Hibernia Bank in San Francisco and Patty was taped on the bank's cameras brandishing an automatic weapon. She now called herself "Tania," and her new personality was wanted for armed robbery.

The follow up $4 million food giveaway was cancelled and, thanks to Jones, the Hearst's initial promise of $6 million may have been reduced to only $1 or 2 million, with Jones receiving all of it in either food or cash.

Patty had been subjected to the most sophisticated brainwashing techniques known, including sensory derivation—tied and blindfolded in a closet for fifty-seven days.

The original plan was to brainwash Patty Hearst as a "Manchurian Candidate" to possibly kill her father, but they fell short of that goal. According to **MK ULTRA** psychologists who later testified at Patty's trial, she had been brainwashed into a state of dissociative disorder, rather than full dissociative identity disorder or DID as it is called. In layman's terms, she did not suffer from amnesia, Her new personality still remembered her old one. Her brainwashing was not complete.

On February 20, 1975, an amateur ham radio operator monitored a communication from Jonestown, Guyana to an undisclosed location in California in which the sender reminded the California receiver to wish Patty Hearst a "Happy Birthday." The next day, the radio operator reported it to the FBI after learning from news reports that, in fact, it was Patty's birthday. Apparently, Jonestown was in communications with the SLA kidnappers.

After the robbery, the group hid out in a rented house in a poor Los Angeles neighborhood where Defreeze ordered Patty and Bill and Emily Harris on a mission to shoplift warm winter clothing and meet him in a motel room in Anaheim. Patty drove the getaway car, but the theft went badly and she had to open fire on a security guard who was chasing after the Harrises. When they arrived at the motel room and turned on the television, they witnessed news reports of the burning of their L.A. hideout. The Los Angeles Police Department went wild. Five hundred LAPD officers fired thousands of rounds of ammunition and dozens of fire bombs into the house. Presumably, DeFreeze was inside and killed, but the body was never clearly identified. The remains, said to be DeFreeze were sent back to his family in Ohio, but identification was impossible because the badly-burned corpse arrived without fingertips or a **head**. Obviously, DeFreeze knew that Patty and the Harrises would be traveling to a cold climate. He also knew that the cost of the motel room was almost as great as the cost of the clothing stolen, but what about the police? Supposedly, they did not know if Patty was in the house when they destroyed it. The Harrises and Patty then travel across country where they hid out in the sparsely populated hills of the southern tier of New York and northern Pennsylvania.

Eventually, Patty, the Harrises and the remaining SLA members reunited in Sacramento, California where they robbed the Crocker National Bank. Patty drove the getaway car. During the holdup, a forty-two year old mother of four was shot and killed and now Patty, or rather "Tania" was wanted for murder.

The group returned to San Francisco where, acting on an anonymous tip, the police arrested Patty Hearst and the Harrises. Jones financed the Harris's defense, but Patty was on her own and sentenced to seven years in prison. Congressman Leo Ryan came to her defense when he organized a congressional petition that was the deciding factor in President Carter's executive order commuting her sentence to just the two years served.

The extraordinary story of Patty Hearst was just a diversion that monopolized the headlines for over a year, that would have read CIA involvement in Watergate had it not been for Patty Hearst. She later recalled to the press, "I think I was very much a distraction from what was going on in Washington. At the time, there was Watergate and we were loosing a president quickly..." Of all the media, **The San Francisco Examiner** had the largest stake in the game. The owner, publisher and editor was Patty's father. His lead investigator was reporter Tim Reiterman who arguably knew more about Patty Hearst's odyssey than anyone else in the world. In preparing for Ryan's visit to Guyana, the CIA, through Gordon Lindsay, specifically requested that Reiterman accompany the congressman. It would appear that Reiterman was targeted for assassination at the airstrip, but he was only wounded and survived. Even professional assassins make mistakes in the fog of war.

The only person to benefit from Patty Hearst's kidnapping was Jim Jones. He put her in prison and Congressman Leo Ryan championed her released. Whether Ryan realized it or not, this was his first encounter with Jones. His second encounter would take his life.

# E I G H T T E E N

## THE ASSASSINATION OF MARTIN LUTHER KING, JR.

*"Everything that we see is a shadow cast by that which we do not see."*

**—Martin Luther King, Civil Rights Leader and Nobel Peace Laureate.**

There is some indication that the CIA killed Martin Luther King, but there is every indication that their asset, Jim Jones, tried to cover it up. If the CIA did kill King, it was probably not for reasons that first come to mind. At the time, there were two opposing factions in the black community: on one side was King's philosophy of peace, understanding, and integration, and on the other side was the violent, revolutionary teachings of Malcolm X and the Black Panthers. Like the FBI, the CIA did not like King, but for reasons of national security, they had a vested interest in King's side winning the debate, but there was a problem. King was a womanizer and "psychologically maladjusted", a fact that even King did not dispute. Many times in his career, he publicly attributed his skills in leadership and creativity to his psychological abnormalities. It was only a matter of time before he and his message were totally discredited. King's death would freeze his philosophy in time and guarantee it would live on in perpetuity. In the words of Mark Twain, "Martyrdom hides a multitude of sins."

In the iconic photograph taken immediately after the assassination, King lay dead on the balcony of his motel room, while three of his aides pointed in the direction of the gunshots; a fourth man, Marrell McCollough, knelt over King's body. McCollough had joined King's entourage just three weeks earlier and vanished immediately afterwards. He was a provocateur working for a federal intelligence agency and on loan to the Memphis Police Department to monitor King's activities. Six years later, he was identified as a CIA operative which poses questions. Was he working for the CIA six years earlier? Was he caring for the fallen leader or just making certain that he was dead?

Allegedly the shots were fired from an open window in the communal bathroom of a boarding house on the other side of a ravine from the motel, and this has always been troubling. The shooter, standing in a bath tub with a rifle out the window, had no assurance that his sniper's nest would not be discovered at any moment in the bathroom that served all the residents on that floor. He had a short window of opportunity, perhaps only a few minutes. How did he know that King was staying in that particular room? The evening before, someone who identified himself as an aide to King phoned the motel manager to request that King's room assignment be changed, and it was. How did the shooter know that King would venture out onto the balcony at precisely the right time. King could have stayed in that room for days and never once gone out onto the balcony, and the shooter had only moments of privacy. This implies collusion with someone inside King's room.

James Earl Ray had escaped from Missouri State Penitentiary the year before and hid out in Mexico. He returned to the US and traveled to Memphis. Somewhere along the way, he met a mysterious man identified only as "Raul" who gave Ray money to check into the boarding house, buy a rifle and a new Ford Mustang car. Ray was shopping for that car when King was assassinated. A rifle, wrapped in newspaper, was found on the sidewalk outside the boarding house. It was never positively identified as either the murder weapon or belonging to Ray, but that was the authority's story and they were sticking to it. Ray was arrested and pleaded innocent, but after considerable police interrogation, admitted to killing King. Ray was tried, convicted, and sentenced. Back in prison, he recanted his confession, claiming to have been coerced into making it. In 1977, Ray once again escaped, this time from Brushy Mountain State Penitentiary, with the help of fellow inmate "Larry" Ed Hacker, who masterminded the escape, but remained behind to be released under an early parole from Tennessee Governor Ray Blanton.

Ray supposedly fled to South American but he would have needed help to secure a fake passport (actually two fake passports). Since he was alone and spoke only English, his logical destination would have been Guyana, the only South American country where English is the official language. Eventually, he flew to England where he stayed until traveling to Portugal and then back to England. He purchased a plane ticket to Belgium but was recognized at Heathrow Airport as he attempted to board the flight. He was arrested and extradited to the US. Aside from traveling under an assumed name, Ray's actions were not those of a fugitive fleeing from the law, but of a tourist on an extended vacation.

One month after Jonestown's White Night, the FBI arrested Governor Ray Blanton and several of his aides for extortion and selling paroles. Named in the indictment was "Larry" Ed Hacker.

This whole adventure was very expensive, but none of the characters had any money. How did Ray travel to Mexico and back, check into the boarding house, buy a rifle and an expensive sports car, then travel to South America, England, Portugal and almost Belgium? Where did Hacker get the money to bribe Governor Blanton? Both Hacker and Ray were prisoners with not a penny in their pockets. The mysterious "Raul" may have had money, but that does not resolve the question of who paid for all this? Obviously, it was someone yet unnamed.

This chapter is not about James Earl Ray, it is about Ray's boarding house landlady, Grace Walden, who sometimes used the name Grace Walden Stevens, after her common law husband. Immediately after King's assassination, Grace Walden claimed that Ray could not have killed King because he was not even in the building at the time; he was out shopping for a car. She said that someone else, who she did not know, was in Ray's room at the time. She told her story to the police, to the press, and anyone who would listen. A few days later, Grace Walden was taken into custody, and supposedly with due process, declared incompetent and remanded to the Tennessee State Prison Mental Hospital, where she would remain, heavily drugged, for the next eight years.

Mark Lane was a nationally recognized attorney and conspiracy theorist who had written or co-written three books on the assassinations of President Kennedy and Martin Luther King. By 1977, Lane had presented sufficient evidence of his conspiracy theories to prompt the House of Representatives to allocate $6 million dollars for an official investigation they entitled, "The House Select Committee on Assassinations" to explore the conspiracies surrounding the murders of King and Kennedy. The hearings were scheduled for November of 1978.

With help from congress, Lane was able to get Grace Walden released from the mental hospital into his custody, but he feared for her life and reportedly sent her to California for safe keeping until her testimony at the Congressional hearings. Where in California was never stated, but as will be apparent later, it might have been in the Peoples Temple.

In the summer of 1978, Lane placed advertisements in newspapers nationwide asking for any information about the assassinations. Temple aide, Terri Buford responded with some very intriguing information about King's death. She promised Lane that Jones knew even more and offered to pay for Lane's trip to Guyana to meet with him. Lane arrived in Jonestown in late summer of 1978 with colleague, Donald Freed, with whom he had co-authored *Executive Action*, a book about the conspiracy to assassinate President Kennedy. Jones reminded the two that he was the recipient of the Martin Luther King Humanitarian of the Year Award and claimed the CIA was out to kill him as well. Lane agreed to represent Jones for a $9,000 per month retainer, paid in advance.

In the aftermath of Jonestown, a memo from Terri Buford to Jones was found in the rubble. It was published in the **New York Times** on December 8, 1978, under the headline, 'Memo Discusses Smuggling Witness into Jonestown'. The memo, titled, 'Confidential—Confidential' reads as follows:

> "Jim I got a message over here that you wanted me to tell Mark Lane that he should look into some alternative means of getting Grace Walden to Guyana ... Do you think that we might ought to offer the tempering of Maxine Swaney's passport ... we have her passport here and it might be something that could be similar to Grace Walden and also if it doesn't look like her, maybe we can swap the picture."

Any information conveniently left behind to be discovered in the rubble of Jonestown is highly suspicious. Did Jones really want to move Grace to her death in Jonestown, or was he trying to hide the fact that she was already there? We may never know if Grace Walden died in Jonestown. She has not surfaced since Mark Lane checked her out of the prison mental hospital. About two weeks before the White Night, Terri Buford left her position as Jones's second in command in Jonestown and traveled to Memphis, Tennessee to move in with Mark Lane. Her trip was seen as a defection from the Peoples Temple, but leaving Jones to move in with his attorney can hardly be seen as a defection. After the mass killings, the FBI wanted to question Jonestown's second-in-command, but Lane refused to surrender her until she was granted full immunity. Buford would live with Lane for many years to come.

Mark Lane had planned to call James Earl Ray and Grace Walden to the stand for the House Hearings. They were his key witnesses and he was denied both. From the onset, the committee declared that Ray would not be allowed to testify because of his prison break. Then they stalled, killing the first day with testimony after testimony from CIA-paid psychiatrists that Grace Walden was not mentally competent to testify. In the middle of their testimony, Lane received a phone call from Jones that Congressman Ryan was in Guyana and Lane's presence was demanded immediately. After a few harsh words to the committee,

Lane stormed out of the hearings, left his assistant in charge, and boarded a flight for Guyana. Without Lane, Ray, or Walden, the hearings fell apart. There was one surprise witness— Marrell McCollough, who never identified himself as a CIA agent, only that back when King was assassinated, he worked for the Memphis Police Department, which was a lie or at least a half truth. McCollough was never on the payroll of the Memphis Police. He worked for army intelligence and was on loan to the FBI, who, working in conjunction with the CIA, assigned McCollough to the Memphis Police. McCollough was not working **for** the police, he was working **with** them, and there is a difference. "For" conjures up images of a common policeman "With" implies an outside consultant, an important fact that the committee never heard or took into consideration when evaluating his testimony. Ultimately, the House Committee determined that there probably was a conspiracy to kill Kennedy and King, but they could not prove it.

King's family, headed by his mother, Alberta, did not believe that Ray had killed Martin. They believed the murder was a conspiracy, orchestrated by the federal government. It took a few years, but eventually the family brought their accusations to a court of law that concluded agencies of the federal government were responsible for the assassination. About this time, in 1974, Alberta King was shot dead while attending services at the Ebenezer Baptist Church in Atlanta. Marcus Wayne Chenault was arrested and convicted of her murder. His behavior in court was nothing short of bizarre. His only concern was whether or not his shots had actually "hit anyone." Chenault was a follower of a Dayton, Ohio black minister, who used the name Rabbi Emmanuel Israel and preached a right-wing doctrine of "Black Hebrew Elitism." The Rabbi had provided Chenault with the gun and transportation to Atlanta. Fearing that he may be implicated, he changed his name to Rabbi Hill and fled the country, along with a thousand of his followers to, of all places, Guyana, where he established a jungle community that he named "Hilltown." This was 1974. The Jonestown site existed, but was occupied by the Shalom Project. It would not be named "Jonestown" for another year. Hilltown actually predated Jonestown. Nothing happened in Guyana without the consent of the CIA. This could have been the subject of Jones's revelations to Mark Lane. James Earl Ray may have been harbored in Hilltown by their leader, who had ordered the death of King's mother.

In the days before, during, and immediately after the assassination of Martin Luther King, there was only one network newsman in Memphis— seasoned NBC reporter, Don Harris. Harris was the only qualified person to independently investigate the crime scene. He conducted many interviews with key witnesses to the killing. His raw data was invaluable and very damning to the government's cover story. Harris's coverage of the racial riots that followed earned him an Emmy Award. Just before the House Assassination Hearings were to convene, NBC News assigned producer/editor Nancy Woodka to accompany Harris back to Memphis to check and recheck his sources and then travel onto Washington for the House Hearings. In the middle of their assignment, Harris was reassigned and ordered to join Congressman Ryan's party for a trip to Guyana and what would be his death. All of his notes, insights, and expertise regarding the killing of Martin Luther King were lost when he was killed at the airstrip and stripped of all of his research.

Greg Robinson, a journalist from the **San Francisco Examiner**, had courageously filmed those same racial riots in Washington, D.C. When the Justice Department demanded his films, he threw them into the Potomac River. Robinson was also killed at the airstrip.

The CIA is its own worst enemy. It starts with a black operation like Jonestown and has some success, so they add another objective to the project. If that looks promising, they add yet another, and so on and so forth, until the cumulative effect of so many of their objectives carried in one basket makes it impossible for them to deny their involvement. In the end, their greed is self-incriminating.

# N I N E T E E N

## THE ADMIRALS

*"MK ULTRA came to my attention early in my tenure as direc-*
*tor of the CIA and I felt it was a warning sign that, if you're not*
*alert, things can go wrong in this organization."*

— Stansfield Turner, retired navy admiral and director of the CIA,
before, during, and after Jonestown, in a documentary entitled,
'Secrets of the CIA.'

At almost every turn in this story, there is a US admiral standing off to one side, quietly directing traffic. No less than three admirals with backgrounds in naval intelligence, participated. The odds of this occurring serendipitously are astronomical. Jonestown was born of a military operation, so it is only understandable that the CIA deferred to military intelligence, that was not under the scrutiny of researchers, conspiracy theorist and politicians, like Leo Ryan, all of whom, were looking over the CIA's shoulder, but none of whom were looking into the activities of military intelligence.

The Office of Naval Intelligence had a long history of sponsoring experiments in mind control. One of their project directors was Dr. Harris Isbel whose work in mental institutions and prisons was funded by the CIA through a grant from the navy. In 1973, Dr. Isbel was summoned to testify to a Senate Committee investigating the CIA's use of human "guinea pigs" in mind altering experiments. The focus of the committee was his use of drugs to reward prisoners for their cooperation. According to Dr. Isbel, volunteers were offered the drug of their choice, even high grade morphine, in exchange for their participation. Dr. Isbel apparently could not understand why the senators were appalled by this navy project, but it did not matter. Once again, Congress was focused on the human rights of the test persons and not on how the experiment results might be used on the general public.

References to the navy start very early in this story. Jones's childhood friend, Dan Mitrione, was ten years Jones's senior. Mitrione spent some of that difference in time working in navy counter intelligence. After Mitrione recruited Jones into the CIA, Jones had to go to "spy school," which he did, at a military base in Honolulu, Hawaii. An obvious choice was Pearl Harbor and the navy. Jones's second foreign assignment was recruiting mercenaries in Brazil, under the direction of Admiral Charles Buford. who was in charge of training Angola-bound mercenaries at a site that would later be known as Jonestown, where Jones's second in command was Buford's daughter, Terri. When Jones's neighbors in Belo Horizonte, Brazil refused to accept that he was a missionary or working for a commercial laundry, Jones lied and said that he was a retired navy officer, but he was too young for that to be true, so he said that he worked for the Office of Naval Intelligence.

Years later, Terri Buford enticed Mark Lane into representing Jones, who single-handedly spoiled Congress's investigation into Martin Luther King's murder. Buford "escaped" Jonestown when she moved into Lane's home. And Lane? He was a former naval intelligence analyst.

After Dr. Lawrence Layton left his post as the director of the US Army's Chemical and Biological Warfare Division, he went to work for the navy. His title was Director of Missile and Satellite Development, but his actual work was top secret and just a continuation of his work with the army. His boss was his neighbor, five star Admiral Chester Nimitz, the pinnacle of the Navy, so revered that a nuclear-powered aircraft carrier was named after him, as well as the headquarters of the Office of Naval Intelligence. Despite his busy schedule, Nimitz took time every day to walk, hand-in-hand, with young Deborah Layton through their neighborhood in the Berkeley Hills. Deborah went on to be the driving force to convince Congressman Ryan to investigate Jonestown, while her brother Larry waited there to kill him.

According to the FBI files on Jonestown, immediately after the deaths, the FBI compiled a list of temple guards suspected of participating in the assault team at the airstrip. The list included: Bob Kice, Tim Kice, Joe Wilson, Albert Touchette, Ron James, Eddy Crenshaw, Ron Tally, and Wesley Bridenbach. The FBI went so far as to obtain a warrant that claimed that these men, "willfully and knowingly did combine, conspire, confederate and agree together with each other and with diverse other unknown persons to kill Leo Ryan." Without explanation, the warrant was suppressed, withdrawn and, even its existence not given any publicity until years later, perhaps due to what happened next.

A man (whose name is redacted from FBI files) reported to the bureau's Dallas, Texas office that he was a retired member of a hunter-killer team working for a government agency whose name was also redacted. A hunter-killer team is basically a sniper squad, in which one man hunts down and identifies a target and the other man kills him. This man reported that he was approached in his home by a current member of the team and two others that he did not know. They asked him to participate in a contract hit in Guyana on who he was told were Red Cross workers accompanied by a news crew. The killing was to be done with assault rifles and a 12 gauge shotgun. Comfortable in his retirement, the man declined the offer. Less than two weeks later, he panicked when he recognized those same three men in news film footage at the airstrip and realized that they had killed a congressman. The FBI took his accusations seriously and set up a sting operation, sending agents, posing as Vietnam veterans into the hunter-killer team. Their only reservations were any discrepancies between what he had told them and what he first reported to Navel Intelligence. Before the man reported his story to law enforcement, he told his story to Navel Intelligence, implying that the hunter-killer team he had worked for was navy. At this point, the FBI dropped their warrant against the temple guards and what follows in their files is 43 blank pages. These pages are not redacted. They are blank, indicating the intelligence was gathered by another agency of the federal government that did not give the FBI permission to release it. This whole incident helps to explain why temple defectors could not identify the assassin who killed Ryan. He may not have been a member of the temple guards. He may have been a navy contract killer. In any event, thirty-five years later, we still do not know who killed Congressman Ryan.

Back when President Ford fired CIA Director William Colby for telling Ryan too much about the agency's work in Angola, he appointed retired Admiral Stansfield Turner to replace him. Admiral Turner had been the president of the Navy's War College. His opening statement about **MK ULTRA** seems out of place because supposedly the program had been shut down five years earlier, but there remained one experiment to combine all the others, and that was Jonestown. Turner took control of the CIA nineteen months before Jonestown's demise. He saw it through to completion and the cover-up that followed, only to leave his post on January 20th, 1981. The date is critical. On that same day, Ronald Reagan was inaugurated president. It appears as if President Reagan's first official act was to fire Turner or perhaps Turner resigned, to pass the torch of silence onto Reagan.

A visit to Congressman Ryan's gravesite at the Golden Gate National Cemetery in San Bruno, California reveals nothing in itself, except that, against all odds, he is buried directly next to none other than Admiral Chester Nimitz. At first this irony might appear to be someone's idea of a sick joke, but after thoughtful consideration, it was a respectful way to put the entire story to rest in one place.

Though it could never be proven in a court of law, the Office of Naval Intelligence was involved and perhaps even responsible for Jonestown.

# T W E N T Y

## DELAYED IRONY

*"Irony cleans away all those secret stains. Irony is the path that leads safely back to official realities."*

—Geoffrey Wall.

Jim Jones was an extremely intelligent sociopath who managed to deceive almost everyone he encountered. He was a brilliant wolf among ignorant sheep. From his followers, to politicians, to the public and even to his CIA employer, Jones enjoyed the feeling of superiority he felt by fouling them all. As serious and cold hearted as he was, he did have a twisted, sarcastic sense of humor, and an extremely odd sense of timing. He told only two running jokes in real time. Terri Buford was in charge of scheduling his sexual relations, so he called her his, "Fucking Secretary." He knew of Lisa Layton's Nazi history and laughingly referred to her as his, "Jewish Nigger." From the beginning, Jones had a sense of his place in history and knew that, one day, historians would look back on his life, so he left them esoteric jokes along the way, jokes that would not become apparent for a very long, pregnant pause.

Early on in Richmond, Indiana, Jones set out to recruit black parishioners to his 'church' by selling them monkeys door-to-door. On the surface, his actions were bizarre, but considering his family's Ku Klux Klan background and his lifelong career to control or even exterminate blacks, selling them monkeys was the ultimate insult, but to Jones, it was a punch line for posterity and just another opportunity to show just how clever he was.

The accepted theory was that Jones moved his followers to Mendocino County, California because an article in *Esquire* magazine that identified it as one of the nine safest places to survive in the event of an all-out nuclear war. Jones told his black followers that he had found their perfect refuge in a cave outside of Redwood Valley. It was just a depression in a cow pasture where grazing cattle would gather around a small fenced in area to take in the cool air from below. A temple member was lowered 150 feet into the vertical shaft, but never found the bottom. Jones continued to tell his followers that this was their life-saving bomb shelter, but failed to tell them the local folklore. Back in the 1800s, a black man allegedly raped a white woman at a nearby stagecoach station and the locals threw him down the hole, which thereafter was known as the "Nigger Hole." To receive social security benefits, Jones's elderly black followers had to present themselves only once to the offices of Social Security. Their payments would continue automatically until their death, but a certificate of death could not be issued from the bottom of the "Nigger Hole." Jones would help them apply, sign their benefits over to him and then just throw them down the hole.

Later, in San Francisco, Jones lead his followers on a protest march to support the erection of anti-suicide fences on the Golden Gate Bridge. Too many people were killing themselves by jumping off the bridge and Jones, who portrayed himself as a humanitarian, demanded that the deaths be prevented. The barriers were built, and for his efforts, Jones received The Martin Luther King Humanitarian of the Year Award. In retrospect, as Jones intended, here was a man who almost single-handedly destroyed Congress's official investigation into King's murder and ordered the largest mass suicide in history. He knew exactly what he was doing. He was playing a joke on history.

Fifteen years after Jones sent a cosmetic double into the Westlake theater to establish a false identity and ten years after this arrest was made public, new evidence of Jones's sinister mind emerged. Cross referencing the arrest date and time with the **Los Angeles Times** entertainment section, revealed that the only movie shown that day was *Jesus Christ Superstar.* Since the police stake-out was ongoing, Jones could have selected any day and movie, but this supposedly Christian preacher elected to have his double masturbate at a showing of *Jesus Christ Superstar*, an irony that would not be played out until a decade and a half later. That is how long-term Jones thought.

Two or three months before Jonestown's demise, the CIA instructed Jones to produce a video to document Jonestown in order to convince the Venezuelans not to invade Guyana's territory, lest they suffer reprisal from the US. One month before Jonestown's demise, Guyana Prime Minister Forbes Burnham invited Venezuelan President Carlos Perez for an official state visit for one and only one purpose; to show him Jones's video in order to convince him to drop Venezuela's land claim and it succeeded. Jones personally conducted the very professional video tour and could not resist injecting his own sense of history into the film that he knew would survive. With the camera following Jones through the pantry of the 'Jonestown Experimental and Herbal Kitchen,' he made a point to say, "Here we have black-eyed peas and rice" (the staple diet of poor blacks), "over here we have cookies" (the means to administer the drugs) "and over here we have Kool-Aid." At this point in time, no one knew the significance of Kool-Aid, but one month later, the world would know. Once again, Jones planted another irony to show off his superior intellect to posterity.

After meeting Josep Mengele in South America, Jones returned to the states and renamed his organization "The Peoples Temple" which sounds more Jewish than the Christian church it was supposed to be. Jones had learned from Mengele that the Nazis used the wealth of the Jews to finance their extermination and he was impressed by the irony so he set out to repeat it by buying former Jewish synagogues, first in Indianapolis and later in San Francisco and Los Angeles. There were few Jewish synagogues for sale in the real estate market. Jones had to work hard to seek them out which shows how important it was for him to emulate the Nazis in his preparations to continue their ethnic cleansing. He was trying to draw as many parallels as possible between the first holocaust and the second that he was planning.

By selecting the same site for Jonestown that the British had proposed to relocate European Jews at the end of World War II, once again, Jones showed his sense of history.

Jones needed a doctor for his experiments and could have financed anyone through medical school, but he selected Larry Schacht, whose namesake, Dr. Hjalmar Horace Greely Schacht was the foremost financier of I. G. Farben and the Nazi's rise to power and the one who coined the phrase over the gates to the Auschwitz Concentration Camp, " And Work Shall Set You Free."

Jones could have named the final event anything, but years earlier, he called it "The White Night." He planned for the suicide/murders to take place on the fortieth anniversary of "The Crystal Night." To start the second holocaust, he emulated the first.

Over Jones's simple Adirondack throne in the Jonestown pavilion hung a sign that read, " Those who do not remember the past are condemned to repeat it. That quote, from philosopher George Santayana is etched in the memorial to the victims of the first holocaust at the Dachau Concentration Camp. The original quote was…"condemned to relive it", but since his followers had not lived through the first holocaust, he altered the quote to "repeat it."

Jones took great pride in deceiving everyone he encountered. Obviously, he could not tell anyone what he was really doing, but his ego was so strong that he had to brag to someone so he left ironic clues in his wake, confident that one day in the future, someone would look back and recognize just how clever he was.

# TWENTY-ONE

## ANNIVERSARIES

*"Are there memories left that are safe from the clutches of phony anniversaries?"*

**—Pope Paul VI.**

It is human nature to celebrate anniversaries. Individuals celebrate birthdays and wedding anniversaries. Nations celebrate holidays. What would the United States be without the Forth of July, Memorial Day, or Labor Day? What would religion be without Christmas, Easter, Passover, or Ramadan. Everyone celebrates anniversaries and the Nazis are no exception, but their celebrations cannot be public displays for obvious reasons. As we have seen, Jones scheduled his White Night to commemorate the fortieth anniversary of the Crystal Night, but the Crystal Night was itself the twentieth anniversary of the signing of the Treaty of Versailles that ended World War I. The treaty signed at the eleventh hour, of the eleventh day, of the eleventh month, imposed such harsh war reparations on Germany that it plunged the country into an unbearable economic depression. Germany's poor were so destitute that they had to strip the wallpaper from their rooms to lick the paste that had been made from a mixture of flour and water. Into this dire situation arose a false hero, who promised to restore Germany's national pride and power. That false hero was Adolph Hitler.

Hitler's master plan called for "A Thousand Year Reich," with the first 120 years devoted to purifying the human race, a plan that, within the minds of some very powerful people, still exists today.

Jonestown was not the only project to culminate in 1978 that had its origins in Operation Paperclip and its supervision under Dr. Lawrence Layton; enter Dr. Erich Traub.

During World War I, Dr. Traub was a captain in the German army and their expert in infectious animal diseases, especially in horses. His work was critical to the German war effort because most of the artillery, supplies, and troops of their enemies were moved by horse power. Kill your enemy's horses and you have effectively killed their movement. Dr. Traub worked in isolation in a laboratory on the island of Insel Riems in the Baltic Sea, where he attempted to perfect the ultimate equine weapon— the bacterium *Burkholderia Mallei* that produces a fatal condition called "Glanders." *Burkholdia Mallei* is classified as a zoonotic agent, in other words, it can be transmittable to humans. Glanders is rampant in the Middle East and Africa, but the last case in the United States was reported in the significant year of 1945.

Between World War I and II, Traub immigrated to the United States where he worked on viruses and bacterium for the Rockefeller Institute, at Princeton University. The Nazis were not yet our enemy, so there was no need for Traub to hide his true affiliations. He was a member of the Amerika Deutscher Volksbund, a German-American club and the headquarters of the American Nazi Party. On weekends, they would gather, 40,000 strong, to march in the streets of New York City, singing Nazi songs, carrying swastika flags, and burning effigies of US Jewish congressmen.

The bacterium that causes Glanders is highly contagious to humans and Traub convinced the US army that it had promise as a bacterial weapon and together with the USDA, they developed the Animal Disease Research Laboratory on Plum Island, off the end of Long Island in New York. The top secret facility was selected because the prevailing winds would blow any contaminants safely out to sea. As the director of the army's Chemical and Biological Warfare Division, Dr. Lawrence Layton was in charge of the Fort Detrick lab in Maryland, the Dugway Proving Grounds in Utah, and the Animal Disease Research Lab on Plum Island, in New York. Dr. Layton was Dr. Traub's superior.

Plum Island is almost as close to Connecticut as it is to Long Island. All of Traub's lab workers commuted by water; some to Long Island, some to Connecticut. The water shuttle to Connecticut docked at the closet landfall in a small village at the mouth of a river.

Traub researched animal diseases that could be transmitted to humans. Even mosquitoes had potential as a weapon of war because they transmit malaria, Dengue fever, and West Nile virus, but in the end, he hit upon something brand new, something unknown to science, something that was carried by the common tick. If you have ever seen a tick, you were probably looking at an adult. In the nymph stage, a tick is so small and transparent that it is almost invisible, yet still capable of transmitting disease.

In 1978, Traub's pet project somehow escaped Plum Island and landed on the shores of Connecticut. The ticks quickly infected wildlife and humans and spread like wildfire throughout the Northeast. The disease was first reported in that little river port village, and since it was new to science and had no name, they named it after that village. The village is South Lyme, Connecticut. The disease is Lyme Disease.

As of this writing in 2013, the US federal government is doing something unthinkable. Without good reason, they have closed the Plum Island animal disease laboratory and moved the entire operation to central Kansas. To locate such a volatile, potentially catastrophic facility upwind of half the US population is beyond stupidity and into the realm of insanity.

There may be other reasons why 1978 was such a banner year for Operation Paperclip experiments. It could have been a passing of the baton; a changing of the guard. Most of the Paperclip scientists who were recruited by the US in 1945 were in their early thirties at the time. By 1978, they had reached retirement age, and if their dreams of purifying the human race in 120 years were to succeed, they had to pass it on to the next generation or at least, "publish" their findings. Dr. Traub chose to "publish before he perished." Mengele and the **MK ULTRA** scientists passed their knowledge onto Jim Jones.

The Nazi's plan to purify the human race that began in 1938, is still active today. Just as the Crystal Night ushered in the First Holocaust, the White Night ushered in the Second Holocaust. Using the Biblical timeframe of forty years for the productive life of a generation, there would need to be two transitions of power, one in November of 1978 and another in November of 2018. They are learning from their mistakes and refining their techniques. AIDS accomplishes the same goals as the concentration camps at less expense, greater effectiveness, and with absolutely no chance of being caught. There are no gas chambers or crematoriums or other physical evidence to point to, but the end result is the same. The unwanted people of the world are being killed off en masse. The first holocaust claimed seven million lives. This second holocaust has so far claimed over thirty-five million lives with a projected one hundred million dead by the next transition in 2018 and it remains to be seen how many millions or billions will be eliminated in the next forty year phase.

# TWENTY-TWO

## NOT THE CONCLUSION

*"You are entitled to your own opinions, but you are <u>not</u> entitled to your own facts"*

**—Senator Daniel Patrick Moynihan.**

What has been presented here are the facts. Together they tell the story you have just read. As disturbing as this book is, it is true. If you choose to believe something else, you are in denial of history.

How could human beings be so evil? The answer is simple. Evil people do not know they are evil. Adolph Hitler thought he was a nice man. He liked children and dogs and brought Germany from the depths of depression to a renewed sense of prominence in the world. Jim Jones was the same. Back in Redwood Valley, he invented a wheelchair-like device for three legged dogs. A photograph of Jones and the dog in the wheelchair has survived. The fact that he had to first amputate a German Sheppard's leg to create a subject for his experiment, was of no consequence to him. To Jones, he was a humanitarian, doing a good deed. In his own twisted way, he thought he was a hero, saving mankind from the yoke of overpopulation. He single-handedly set out on a quest to eliminate those he considered to be the unwanted people of the world in order to correct the famine, water shortages, global warming, and wars that are caused by just too many people on this planet. Scientists like Dr. Lawrence Layton are the worst justifiers. They believe that, if something **can** be done, it **should** be done. Morality never gets in the way of their pursuit of science.

The real United States of America is no more than the un-elected, invisible government of the Central Intelligence Agency. Congress is just a group of argumentative egotists with nice hair who spend most of their time soliciting contributions from special interest groups or on the phone with their brokers buying stock in companies they have just given lucrative government contracts to. It is called "insider trading" and supposedly illegal, but rampant in the halls of Congress. Congressmen are more likely to be embroiled in a scandal over sex or money, than to accomplish anything of value. Even when

151

they are "working" in session, they spend about a third of their time berating each other, in a scene that is closer to an eighth grade school recess than a viable government. Congressmen, who truly want to make a difference for their constituents, like Leo Ryan, are rare. The Judicial branch sits in their chairs waiting for someone to ask them a question. Even though their answers may be correct, their's is not a proactive government. The true power of the US federal government lies in the Executive branch where presidents and their administrations come and go, but the CIA goes on ad infinitum and the CIA is broken beyond repair. It took over thirty years to uncover what they were doing in Jonestown. Are Americans willing to wait another thirty years to uncover what they are doing today?

It is very telling that the CIA spends half of their annual budget on disinformation campaigns. To put that into perspective: they spend half of their taxpayer-funded budget on such objectionable activities as to require them to spend the other half to hide those activities from the general public and the taxpayers who support them.

Currently, the news is full of stories about terrorist cells and sleeper cells, but nowhere are there more clandestine cells than in the hallways of CIA headquarters that boast the longest corridor in the world, with door after endless, unidentified door, behind which are held secret projects that are not shared with even the office next door. Their system of compartmentalized knowledge on a need to know basis is what allowed Jonestown to happen unabated, but it was just the tip of the **MK ULTRA** iceberg. The CIA conducted hundreds of macabre medical experiments on thousands of unwitting American citizens without regard to the adverse physical and mental effects inflicted on the test persons. Call it a "renegade faction," call it "misguided intentions," call it "Nazi infiltration," call it whatever you want, but do not lose sight of the fact that it was all the CIA.

We need to recognize and accept that the the CIA has not represented American values for decades. They financed Fidel Castro and then backed a failed invasion to overthrow him. They supported UNITA in Angola that eventually lost. Angola's rich oil reserves now go to supply over twenty-five percent of China's needs. They supported Forbes Burnham in Guyana, but in the end, communist Cheddi Jagan took power; the same Chaddi Jagan that Jim Jones had opposed in the early 1960's. They failed to foretell the collapse of communism in Eastern Europe. The fall of the Berlin Wall and the Soviet Union came as a complete surprise to what supposedly is the premier intelligence agency in the world. In Afghanistan, the CIA provided money and arms to the

Mujahideen, who evolved into the Taliban and Al-Quaeda, and used **our** weapons to kill **our** soldiers. The US has entrusted its security to an agency that was totally blind to the terrorist attacks on 9/11.

Currently, the US is winding down a protracted war in Iraq that cost billions of dollars and thousands of American lives; but why? In the very beginning, there was one, and only one, newscast that Prime Minister Saddam Hussein had ordered the invasion of Kuwait because the US was using a new technique to horizontally drill under the border and steal his oil. The story was immediately censored in the US and never heard again. President, and former CIA Director, George H. Bush and his oil company friends, along with their Kuwaiti partners, were using the new technology to establish well heads in Kuwait to drill down and then sideways under the border horizontally to illegally extract oil that belonged to Iraq. Hussein had no choice but to invade Kuwait, capture the well heads, and stop the bleeding. Bush ordered American troops into harm's way to drive the Iraqis back to Baghdad, but no further. He knew Hussein was right. In their retreat, the Iraqis set the well heads on fire. When Bush's son was elected president, the CIA failed to inform him of their crimes against Hussein, choosing instead to vilify him as a threat to the US because they claimed he had, "Weapons of Mass Destruction"— a catchy sound bite, but a total lie. The new President Bush ordered another invasion of Iraq, this time killing Hussein and his sons, whose only crime against the US was defending their property. Behind this total fiasco, was the CIA feeding false information to Washington to cover up the US elite's theft of millions of dollars in oil.

The CIA has not gotten anything right in decades. Its defense has always been that the public only sees their failures and not their successes. Thier successes may be invisible because they do not exist. There is a disconnection between the CIA and the government it is supposed to represent. At least the communists spread communism. The CIA, on the other hand, does not spread democracy; it is too messy. It prefers to back dictators or military regimes that are easier to control. Today, the CIA is sixty-seven years old and it is time to reevaluate. Originally, it was conceived as a passive agency to gather intelligence that has evolved into an active killing machine for the federal government. Traditional warfare of advancing armies gaining ground is a thing of the past. Our soldiers are being replaced by strategic surgical strikes by CIA surveillance and attack drones. The CIA already has the authority to use its drones to kill American citizens in foreign countries, not for what they have done, but for what the CIA perceives they might do in the future. The present debate in Washington is whether this license to kill Americans includes Americans on American soil. Considering their history, can The CIA be trusted with such a critical role? If the US is to carry forward with any amount of humanity and civility, the CIA needs to be totally revamped. It happened once before, at the end of World War II, when the gentlemen's club at the OSS was disbanded and replaced with the hard-nosed CIA to fight the Cold War, but the Cold War is over and the CIA has outlived that purpose. What is it doing with its $55 billion dollar annual "black budget," other than creating animosity and hatred of Americans around the world? Presently, most intelligence is gathered electronically by the National Security Agency, the National Reconnaissance Office, and military intelligence. "Boots on the ground" are provided by Homeland Security and the FBI. So, what is the CIA doing? They say they are protecting the US from its enemies, but what they will not say is that their activities around the world are largely responsible for creating those enemies. They are suspiciously silent. Like rowdy children playing quietly in the next room, you can be reasonably assured that they are drawing on the walls with crayons.

The CIA is not inherently evil. They are like anything else in this world; they have good people and bad people, though their bad people are generally more ruthless and mean-spirited than most. The difference is, with their power, resources, contacts, and relative immunity from prosecution, the bad people can inflict a tremendous amount of damage. This was the case with Jim Jones, whose legacy has left nothing but death and destruction in its path.

Because of Jones's work, the nation's mentally ill are dying homeless on the streets, languishing in prison, or firing assault weapons on school yards full of children. AIDS is running rampant throughout the prison system, the gay community, and among the estimated one million American heroin addicts. The demographic that is suffering the fastest spread of the virus is young black people, ages 13 through 24, due largely to laws the majority of our states have enacted. In thirty-nine states, it is a felony to knowingly transmit HIV or even to fail to inform a sexual partner, whether that partner actually contracts the virus or not. Violators are labeled "sex offenders" and sentenced to anywhere from 10 to 25 years in prison, a life sentence for anyone with HIV. These supposedly well-intentioned laws have only served to drive the problem underground by discouraging young people from being tested. If they do not know they are HIV positive, and they infect someone, they have not broken the law. Rather than commit to a celibate life or risk prison, they choose instead to live in ignorance and it is that ignorance that is perpetuating the epidemic and dooming the next generation of black Americans.

Do not be mislead by the plethora of propaganda. **AIDS is a viral weapon in an undeclared war of ethnic cleansing.** In the US, blacks and homosexuals are fifteen times more likely to contract AIDS than whites. Taken separately, the black population in the US has the same rate of infection as a sub-Saharan African country. The death rate from AIDS in blacks worldwide is approaching their birth rate, after which fewer and fewer black people will inhabit this earth, until they are totally annihilated. Whether this was created by Nazis working within the CIA or Jim Jones working in the CIA or some combination of the three, whether you applaud their actions or abhor their actions, regardless of who is responsible or how you feel about it, recognize this episode in history for what it really is: **The Second Holocaust**, because if you do not, you will be totally blind to the **Third**, and the next time, **they may be coming for you!**

# WORKS REFERENCED

Portions of the Preface are the author's personal life experience. Chapter Five is based on historical facts, but entirely the author's artistic license. The rest of this book may be referenced and confirmed in the following works by others for those willing to spend years of digging to uncover the truth about Jonestown and the creation of the AIDS epidemic. Any one piece of this puzzle is not compelling but taken together, all the pieces reveal the picture; the known history and the story you have just read.

## BOOKS
Cantwell, Alan, Jr. M.D. *AIDS: The Mystery & The Solution.* Los Angeles, CA.: Aries Rising Press, 1984.

Cantwell, Alan, Jr. M.D. *AIDS And the Doctors of Death: An Inquiry into the Origin of the AIDS Epidemic.* Los Angeles, CA. :Aries Rising Press, 1988.

Beckford, James A. *Cult Controversies: The Societal Response to New Religious Movements.* London: Tavistock Publications, Ltd., 1985.

Brown, Raymond Keith. *AIDS, Cancer and the Medical Establishment.* New York: Robert Speller Publishers, 1986.

Douglass, William Campbell, M.D. *The Greatest Biological Disaster in the History of Mankind: AIDS: The End of Civilization.* Clayton, GA.: Valet Publishers/ Tri-State Press, 1989.

Duesberg, Peter H. *Inventing the AIDS virus.* Washington, D.C.: Regnery Publishing, Inc., 1996.

Feisod, Ethan. *Awake in a Nightmare: Jonestown; The Only Eyewitness Account.* New York, London : W.W. Norton and Company, 1981.

Kerns, Phil with Dough Wead. *People's Temple- People's Tomb.* Plainfield, N.J.: Logos International, 1979.

Killduff, Marshall and Ron Javers. *The Suicide Cult: The Inside Story of the Peoples Temple Sect and the Massacre in Guyana.* New York: Bantam Books, Inc.,1978.

Klineman, George Sherman Butler and David Conn with research by Anthony O. Miller.
*The Cult that Died: The Tragedy of Jim Jones and the Peoples Temple.* New York: G.P. Putnam's sons, 1980.

Krause, Charles A. with Lawrence M. Stern, Richard Harwood and the staff of the *Washington Post. Guyana Massacre: The Eyewitness Account.* New York: Berkeley Publishing Corporation, 1978.

Lane, Mark. *The Strongest Poison. New York*: Hawthorne Books; a division of Elsevier-Dutton, 1980.

Langguth, A. J. *Hidden Terrors: The Truth About U.S. Police Operations in Latin America.* New York: Pantheon Books, 1978. (A good source of information about Dan Mitrione's CIA career).

Layton, Deborah. *Seductive Poison: A Jonestown Survivor's Story of Life and Death in the People's Temple.* New York: Doubleday / Anchor Books, 1998.

Levi, Ken. *Violence and Religious Commitment: Implications of Jim Jones's People's Temple Movement.* University Park, PA. and London: The Pennsylvania State University Press, 1982.

Maguire, John and Mary Lee Dunn. *Hold Hands and Die: The Incredible True Story of the People's Temple, Reverend Jim Jones, and the Tragedy in Guyana.* New York: Dale Books, 1978.

Meiers, Michael. *Was Jonestown a CIA Medical Experiment? A Review of the Evidence.*
Lewiston, New York, Queenston, Canada and Lampeter, Whales: The Edwin Mellen Press, 1989.

Mills, Jeanne. *Six Years with God: Life Inside Reverend Jim Jones's People's Temple.* New York: A & W Publishers, Inc., 1979.

Moore, Rebecca. *A Sympathetic History of Jonestown: The Moore Family Involvement in*
*Peoples Temple.* Lewiston, New York: The Edwin Mellon Press, 1985.

Moore, Rebecca. *The Jonestown Letters: Correspondence of the Moore Family 1970-1985.* Lewiston, New York: The Edwin Mellon Press, 1985.

Naipaul, Shiva. *Journey to Nowhere: A New World Tragedy.* New York and Middlesex, England: Penguin Books, 1982. First published in Great Britain in 1980, under the title: *Black and White.*

Nugent, John Peer. *White Night: The Untold Story of What Happened Before and Beyond Jonestown.* New York: Rawson, Wade Publishers, Inc., 1979.

Olsen, Paul R.. *The Bible Said it Would Happen.* Minneapolis, MN: Ark Books, 1979.

Ostrander, Sheila and Lynne Schroeder. *Psychic Discoveries Behind the Iron Curtain.*
Englewood Cliffs, NJ: Prentice-Hall , Inc., 1970. Republished by Bantam Books in 1971.

Posner, Gerald L. and John Ware. *Mengele: The Complete Story.* New York: Cooper Square Press, 1986.

Powers, Thomas. *The Man Who Kept the Secrets: Richard Helms and the CIA.* New York: Pocket Books, a division of Simon and Schuster, 1979.

Reiterman, Tim with John Jacobs. *Raven: The Untold Story of Rev. Jim Jones and His People.* New York: E. P. Dutton, Inc., 1982.

Reston, James, Jr. *Our Father Who Art in Hell.* New York: Times Books, a division of Quadrangle/ The New York Times Book Co., Inc., 1981.

Rubenstein, Richard R. *The Cunning of History: The Holocaust and the American Future.* New York: Harper and Row Publishers, Inc., 1975.

Scheeres, Julia. *A Thousand Lives: The Untold Story of Hope, Deception, and Survival at Jonestown.* New York: Free Press, 2011.

Shirer, William L. *The Rise and Fall of the Third Reich: A History of Nazi Germany.*
New York: Fawcett Crest Books, a unit of CBS Publications, 1959.

Shilts, Randy. *The Mayor of Castro Street: The Life and Times of Harvey Milk.* New York: St. Martin's Press, 1982.

Speer, Albert. *Inside the Third Reich.* New York: Collier Books, a division of Macmillan Publishing Co., Inc., 1970.

Stockwell, John. *In Search of Enemies: A CIA Story.* New York: W.W. Norton, 1978.

Targ, Russell and Keith Harary. *The Mind Race: Understanding and Using Psychic Abilities.* New York: Villard Books, 1984.

Theilmann, Bonnie with Dean Merrill. *The Broken God.* Elgin, IL: David C. Cook Publishing Co., 1979.

Timberg, Craig and Daniel Halperin, Ph.D. *Tinderbox: How the West Sparked the AIDS Epidemic and How the World Can Finally Overcome It.* New York: Penguin Press, 2012.

Weightman, Judith Mary. *Making Sense of the Jonestown Suicides: A Sociological History of Peoples Temple.* New York and Toronto: The Edwin Mellon Press, 1983.

Weinberg, David Jay. *Mengele's Legacy.* Danbury, CT: Rutledge Books, Inc., 2001.

White, Mel. *Deceived.* Old Tappan, NJ: Fleming H. Revell / Spire, 1979.

Wise, David and Thomas B. Ross, *The Invisible Government.* New York: Vintage Books, a division of Random House, 1964.

Wooden, Kenneth. *The Children of Jonestown.* New York: McGraw-Hill Book Co., 1981.

Yee, Min S. and Thomas Layton. *In My Father's House: The Story of the Layton Family*
*and the Reverend Jim Jones.* New York: Holt Rinehart, and Winston, 1981. Republished by Berkley Books in 1982.

## MAGAZINE ARTICLES

Bird, Caroline. "Nine Places to Hide." *Esquire Magazine* January, 1962. pp. 55-132.

Brown, Michael H. "Mind over Matter." *Reader's Digest* May, 1981. pp. 113-117.

Harris, William. "New Evidence Reveals Jim Jones Still Alive in Brazil." *Globe* May, 12, 1981. p.35.

Kilduff, Marshal and Phil Tracey. "Inside People's Temple." *New West Magazine* August, 1979. pp. 30-38.

Witten, Martin A. " Guyana: Autopsy of Disbelief." *Lab World* 1979, volume 30, pp. 14-19.

"The Cult of Death." *Newsweek Magazine* December 4, 1978. pp. 38-77.

## NEWSPAPER ARTICLES

The tremendous volume of newspaper articles precludes an itemized listing. Search each paper's archives for details. Newspapers are listed in the order of their contribution to the story.

*The San Francisco Chronicle*
*The San Francisco Examiner*

*The New York Times*
*The Oakland Tribune*
*The San Jose Mercury News*
*The Indianapolis Star*
*The Indianapolis News*
*The Ukiah Daily Journal*
*The Guyana Chronicle*
*The Guyana Graphic*
*The Washington Post*
*The Miami Herald*

## FILMS and TELEVISION

"Guyana: Cult of the Damned."

"The Guyana Tragedy-The Story of Jim Jones." A CBS television docudrama.

"In Search of... Jim Jones."

"The People vs., Dan White" A PBS television docudrama.

"Confessions of Frank Terpil: The Most Dangerous Man in the World." A British Broadcasting Corporation television interview.

"The Times of Harvey Milk." A PBS television documentary.

"Deceived." A Mel White Production, available from Gospel Films, Inc. Box 455, Muskegon, MI. 49443.

"Milk"- An award-winning docudrama about the life of Harvey Milk.

"Bamazon" An Arts and Entertainment television series that offers a rare look into Guyana's mysterious interior.

## MUSEUMS / RESEARCH CENTERS

The Mae Brussels Research Center. A vast storehouse of information on Jonestown, mostly in audio tapes of her radio program, "World Watchers International." <maebrussell.com>.

The San Francisco Historical Society. A excellent source of first-hand accounts of Jim Jones's life in in San Francisco. <sfhistory.org>.

## GOVERNMENT REPORTS

"The Assassination of Representative Leo J. Ryan and the Jonestown, Guyana Tragedy". Report of a Staff Investigative Group to the Committee on Foreign Affairs, U.S. House of Representatives (Washington, D.C.; Government Printing Office, Document #96-223, 96th Congress). This document is difficult to locate because it went out of print almost immediately. It can be found in *Historic Documents of 1979* in the reference section of any well-stocked library.

"Review of the Implication of Recommendations Relating to the Death of Representative Leo J. Ryan". U.S. Congress, House Committee on Foreign Affairs, Subcommittee on International Operations, Washington, D.C., U.S. Government Printing Office, 1980.

"Guyana". Department of State Publication #8095, Washington, U.S. Government Printing Office. Revised in March of 1979, four months after Jonestown. Publication #044-000-91116-7.

FBI Files. The FBI's reading room of information that has been released under the Freedom of Information Act numbers over 50,000 pages of evidence, interviews and reports. It is extremely valuable, but somewhat flawed. The copies were scanned reproductions of originals, but some of those originals were mimeographed and the results are illegible. There are redactions on every page, mostly to conceal names, but often to conceal entire paragraphs or even pages. Following one critical point in the file, when it appears that it is about to reveal who actually shot Ryan, there are forty-three entirely blank pages.
<FBI Reading Room/Vault/ Jim Jones/ rymur.gov.>

CIA Files. As might be expected, the CIA has not released much information in response to FOIA requests. What little the is available may be found at <CIA Reading Room/ Jonestown. gov.>

**INTERNET SIGHTS**

There is a wealth of information on the internet, but one must be cautious. This subject seems to attract religious fanatics, government disinformation campaigns and people trying to justify their involvement but among all that are some very professionally researched reports. The following contributors are recommended as a starting point on an internet journey that might take longer than a lifetime to conclude. Simply search their names.

Dave Emory/ Jonestown

Gerald Posner/ Jonestown

John Judge/ Jonestown

Jim Hougan/ Jonestown

Dr. Alan Cantwell/ AIDS

You Tube/ Jonestown (offers historic film footage, but most is Jones's propaganda.)

**PHOTOGRAPHS**

If a picture really is worth a thousand words, there is an entire, previously untouched, library on this subject in the offices of Bettmann Archives and Getty Imagies. Their photos and videos are displayed on their websites, but back in the early 1980s, I visited the Bettmann Archives New York City headquarters and know they have far more photos than they offer on their website, so to do a thorough search, a visit to both company's headquarters is necessary.

CPSIA information can be obtained at www.ICGtesting.com
Printed in the USA
LVOW12s0103150514

385809LV00005B/9/P

9 781457 525032